PREVENTING
AUTISM&ADHD

PREVENTING
AUTISM&ADHD

Controlling Risk Factors
Before, During and After Pregnancy

Dr. Debby Hamilton, MD, MSPH

HEDWIN PRESS

Library of Congress Cataloging-in-Publishing Data

Preventing Autism & ADHD :
    Controlling risk factors before, during and after pregnancy / Hamilton
    p. cm.
    Includes bibliographical references and index.
    ISBN 978-0-9888204-0-1
    1. Diseases of children and adolescents
Hamilton, Deborah E.

    RJ370-550   2013

Library of Congress Number 2013939151

Hedwin Press, LLC, Louisville, Colorado

ISBN 978-0-9888204-0-1

This book was set in Garamond Adobe Pro by Mark E. Baker.
Cover design by Kristina Ivic.
Printed and bound by Royal Palm Press, Florida

www.HedwinPress.com
Louisville, Colorado

Hedwin Press books are available at special quantity discounts for use as premiums and sales promotions, or for use in training programs. For more information contact Hedwin Press, 812 Pinehurst Ct., Louisville, CO 80027, phone: 303-818-9513, email: mark@hedwinpress.com

First Edition
10 9 8 7 6 5 4 3 2

Includes indexes.

This book is dedicated
to my children,
my patients,
and the health of future children

Note

This book provides the reader with accurate information on the subject matter covered. It is published with the understanding that it does not render medical advice. If medical advice is needed, the reader must consult with a qualified medical professional based upon their individual health situation.

Contents

Part 4: Infancy and Early Childhood Autism & ADHD Prevention

Foreword

Autism may be our most devastating childhood illness. Survival is not the challenge; the challenge becomes facing the loss of their human potential that pulls on our hearts on a daily basis. ADHD makes success in any arena a continual challenge.

We have made huge advances in the treatment of autism and autism spectrum disorders in the last decade. We are now beginning to recognize the interwoven problems that relate to food, digestion, metabolism, and detoxification. In spite of these advances our treatment remains partial and at times quite superficial. Medications do not treat any aspect of the illness. They only minimize specific symptoms. Diet change, nutritional supplements, and biomedical treatments offer more hope, but still these children and these families suffer dearly.

In ADHD, recent reports demonstrate a waning value of stimulant medications. They appear to work wonders in the first few months, but that fades over time and by two years all of the benefits fall away. Additionally, stimulants carry a real risk of addiction, heightened anxiety, weight loss, stunted growth, and personality change. In spite of treatment, children diagnosed with ADHD have significantly higher rates of substance abuse, school failure, relationship struggles, criminal behavior, and job loss. These are life long concerns.

In the last few decades the incidence of these illnesses and most other psychiatric disorders in children have skyrocketed. Depression, pediatric bipolar and other illnesses claim more and more children each year. The percent of affected children is rising in a horrifying fashion. Why? The genetics in this country have not changed appreciably in the last half-century. The change is in the environmental factors that we now know actually manage and direct our genetic code. This new field is called *epigenetics* and it helps to explain why we are facing this epidemic of neurodevelopmental problems including autism ADHD. Quite simply, we now have more additives, heavy metals, persistent organic pollutants, untested industrial chemicals, processed foods, and neuro-endocrine disruptors that we encounter daily. Our diets have been massively compromised. All of this changes our genetic expression and increases the risk for neurodevelopmental problems in our children.

There is good news hidden in this discovery. We can't change our genetic code. But we can alter the epigenetic factors that run our genetic code. This is at the heart of Dr. Hamilton's book. Take control of your environment and take control of your risk factors. We can change what our genetic code expresses by changing the epigenetic influences that we encounter each day. The science that documents these effects is available now.

The deepest wish of any prospective parent sounds something like this: I want a healthy, whole child. While the treatment of both autism and ADHD remains imperfect, the prevention of autism offers clear-eyed hope. Dr. Debby Hamilton's book provides clear and sound advice for any parents considering pregnancy or with a young infant. This becomes particularly important if there is a sibling or close relative on the autism spectrum or challenged by ADHD. Statistically, this increases the risk of having a child identified with a neurodevelopmental disorder at some point in their life.

The key to remember is that statistics speak to the average risk within a population. Dr. Hamilton understands well the nature of risks and the statistics. By providing advice about a range of prenatal and early childhood influences, Dr. Hamilton changes the risk factors that will control your child's destiny.

One factor that has united autism and ADHD in the past is the lack of understanding about cause and the lack of useful strategies for prevention. Well, that is now changing thanks to Dr. Hamilton. An ounce of prevention is worth a pound of cure. Nowhere is this sage observation more accurate than in the prevention and treatment of childhood disorders such as autism and ADHD. I encourage you to take charge of your destiny and, more importantly, to take charge of your child's destiny. We do not have to fall prey to averages and epidemics. We have a pound of prevention within our grasp and that is worth a fortune.

Scott Shannon, MD
Author of Mental Health for the Whole Child, Norton-2013

Preface

This book began with a simple question from mothers: "What can I do to prevent my next child from developing autism and ADHD?" This request came repeatedly from mothers who had one child with autism or ADHD and were concerned about the health of their next child. Since we know that having one child with either of these disorders increases the chance of having any further children with these issues, this was an excellent question. It was also one that I needed to research so I could provide credible answers.

My first clues to understanding the answers to this important question came from experience in my own practice. I have an integrative pediatric practice called *Holistic Pediatric Consulting*, in Boulder, Colorado. Although I see a wide range of children's health issues, my focus is on chronic health conditions such as autism, ADHD, sensory processing issues, emotional issues, allergies, digestive issues, and growth issues. In addition to complicated sick children, I also take care of children with no health issues whose families want an integrative pediatrician for well-child care. As I delved into the health histories of children with chronic health issues versus those with no medical issues, I began to see distinct patterns.

Children in my practice with chronic health issues, especially autism and ADHD, usually have common threads that run through their medical histories, beginning with their mother's and sometimes their father's medical history. I repeatedly saw the multiple toxins that people were exposed to daily from their homes, yards, and consumer products. These families were also consuming nutritionally depleted foods. Their food choices led to children with weaker immune systems with increased infections. Poor nutrition also appeared to contribute to more hormone problems, and more problems processing all of the chemicals from their environment. Finally, the most strikingly consistent finding in these children was that children with health issues usually come from parents with health issues. A mother with health problems seemed especially prone to have a child with chronic illnesses.

In contrast, my well-child families also had some consistent threads running through their families' health histories. I was impressed with the quality of their food. Young children will eat green vegetables and enjoy them. They avoid processed foods and limit sugar intake. Many of their diets were based on organic food or even produce from local farms. As I explored information about their home environments, I was also impressed by their knowledge and concern about the products their family came into contact with on a daily basis. Who knew that there were chemicals in shampoo that acted like estrogen? Just as sick children often come from sick parents, healthy children often come from healthy parents. I found that healthy babies are more likely to come from healthy mothers.

With this clinical information, I knew I needed to understand these correlations. Six years and over six hundred references later, I was able to put my clinical observations together with a solid academic foundation. There is a lot of information on risk factors for autism and ADHD that encompass factors such as diet, digestion, toxins, and genetics. Many of these risk factors relate to the patterns I was seeing in my families so I knew I was onto something.

During the writing of this book, I organized risk factors into a time line that began before pregnancy and continued into the first several years of a child's life. The more I put all of these risk factors in the proper order, the more I realized how critical the time before pregnancy is to having a healthy baby. Since a healthy mother increases the chance of having a healthy baby, we had to get these mothers ready before their bodies are able to optimally support a healthy pregnancy. Ultimately this has led to the before pregnancy part being the longest section of the book, and definitely the most important section to understand for a healthy new child.

✧✧✧

As with most things in life, there is a personal aspect to this story. Along with being a pediatrician for the past twenty years, I have been a mother for over seventeen years. My children have taught me so much about parenting and health. They have also led me in my personal journey from general pediatric practice to nutrition training, public health science, and finally to my own integrative practice. Each of my children has learning issues: one has ADHD and the other has dyslexia (a reading disorder). They are bright and amazing teenagers, but both have suffered because of their learning disabilities. When my daughter was an infant, she also had medical problems with severe colic and poor growth. As their parent, I wanted to do everything to help them. I began with traditional medicine and then explored from there. When I say we tried every type of therapy and supplement, I mean we tried them all. My son was getting acupuncture at age seven and my daughter could tell you that eggs were brain food and let you know if she hadn't taken her "fishy" pills that day (omega-3 fatty acids). After all of my formal education and experience as a mother of children with chronic health issues, I knew how I wanted to practice medicine and the children I wanted to help.

✧✧✧

Since I treat children with autism and ADHD, I need to state that I love working with these children and their families. Trying to prevent children from developing these diseases in no way negates this. I want to prevent the suffering and frustrations that these children encounter on a daily basis, not negate their unique traits and characteristics. I also want to prevent the suffering of families who deal with ongoing daily struggles that impact their entire lives. I wouldn't change my son, although I would like to have made school easier. I wouldn't change my daughter either, but it would have been better if I had known she was allergic to soy and in pain for the first years of her life.

This book reflects all of the wisdom I have gained from my training, my clinical practice, my wonderful families and the hundreds of research articles dedicated to further understanding autism and ADHD.

I wish I could guarantee that following my program will prevent all children from developing autism and ADHD. However, I can guarantee that women and their babies will feel better and have a better chance at avoiding chronic disease. Luckily, there is a lot we already know about the risk factors involved and new information is released every day.

Every child deserves the best possible chance for health. Our country needs to acknowledge our children are increasingly unhealthy in order for people to make changes. These changes need to include pre-conception health programs for women contemplating pregnancy.

Our children are our future. Let's give them the best chance we can, beginning with healthy women having healthy babies.

Debby Hamilton, MD, MSPH

Part 1

Saving Our Children

1

An Epidemic

THE RATES OF AUTISM are rising rapidly. The U.S. Centers for Disease Control and Prevention (CDC) tracks these rates.[1] In 1982, only 1 of 2,222 children were affected. In 2007, people were shocked when the CDC reported that 1 in 150 had autism. And in 2013, the CDC published a report that 1 in 50 were affected (2%).[2] In just six years autism has increased 71%. Autism has gone from a rare disease to one that is increasingly common.

Hundreds of thousands of U.S. children have this terrible disease and about 44,000 children acquire the disease every year. There are more cases of Autism Spectrum Disorder (ASD) than childhood cancer, juvenile diabetes, and pediatric AIDS combined.

Our boys are especially at risk. Autism is much more common in boys with rates of approximately 4 boys for every 1 girl being affected. When breaking these CDC rates down for boys, the situation becomes even more frightening: in 2009, 1 in 58 boys were affected. In 2012, 1 in 32 boys are considered to be on the autism spectrum.[3]

This is a worldwide problem affecting both wealthy and poor countries. England reported in 2006, that 1 in 86 of its children had ASD.[4] South Korea released the statistic in 2011 that 1 in 38 of its children were affected.[5] Many other countries do not formally track their ASD rates, yet they report ever increasing numbers of children with autism.

The CDC uses a multi-state, scientifically valid sampling method to determine autism rates, yet some people argue that increased rates for autism are only because we now more readily diagnose this disease. I find it difficult to believe that physicians today are better diagnosticians by over four thousand percent than their predecessors. Actually, autism is easy to recognize. Behaviors and symptoms such as hand flapping, lack of speech, and poor sociability are obvious. Many non-practitioners recognize ASD easily. In fact, many parents know that there is a serious problem with their child before a practitioner diagnosis is made. The very large rise in autism rates cannot be explained away by improved diagnosis alone.

It now seems like we all know someone touched by autism.

The new 5th Edition of American Psychiatric Association Diagnostic and Statistical Manual of Mental Disorders replaces separate diagnoses of autism, Asperger syndrome, and pervasive developmental disorder not otherwise specified (PDD-NOS) with a single diagnosis of Autism Spectrum Disorder (ASD). According to the CDC, ASDs are "a group of developmental disabilities that can cause significant social, communication and behavioral challenges."
—Individuals with autism exhibit all of the following: (1) deficits in social interaction/communication, (2) restrictive, repetitive patterns of behaviors, interests or activities, (3) symptoms are present in early childhood and (4) symptoms together limit overall functioning.

Note: The term "autism" is used a synonym for the term "ASD" throughout this book.

In addition to autism, millions of families are affected by the neurodevelopmental disease *Attention Deficit Hyperactivity Disorder (ADHD)*. The ADHD rates are tracked by the CDC and have also risen dramatically: up 22% between 2003 and 2007, with estimates of 9.5% of U.S. children affected by this disorder.[6] Again, boys are primarily affected. Approximately 13.2% of boys have some type of ADHD. Nationally, about 1 in 6 children[7] are affected by learning disabilities including autism and ADHD—almost 17% of our children! In a typical classroom of 30 children, 5 will have a learning disability.

There has been debate about how to label the severity of these growing developmental disorders (autism and ADHD). The CDC characterizes autism as only a "public health concern," while it labels obesity as an "epidemic." An epidemic is defined as something that affects a disproportionately large number of individuals within a population, region, or community at the same time. Autism's shadow is falling on more and more children. To me and to others who have studied the rates of autism and ADHD, the spread of these developmental disorders needs to be classified and addressed as an epidemic.

> *The new 5ᵗʰ Edition of American Psychiatric Association Diagnostic and Statistical Manual of Mental Disorders made changes to the definition of ADHD.*
>
> *ADHD is characterized by a pattern of behavior, present in multiple settings (e.g., school and home), that can result in performance issues in social, educational. or work settings. Symptoms are divided into two categories of inattention and hyperactivity/impulsivity that include behaviors such as failure to pay close attention to details, difficulty organizing tasks, excessive talking, fighting, or an inability to remain seated in appropriate situations. Patients must have at least 6 symptoms from the inattention and hyperactivity/impulsivity criteria. Symptoms must present before the age of 12.*

Impacts of the Problem

My own children have struggled with neurologic issues. One of my children has a reading disorder (dyslexia) and the other has ADHD. I can attest to the hours of tutoring, the frustrations of school, and the added financial burden that come with learning and developmental issues. But my struggles have been minor compared to those suffered by families when they have a child with autism.

Having a child with autism completely alters a family's day-to-day life. Every meal can be a battleground trying to convince their child to eat. Parents have long nights of trying to get their child to sleep and then waking up exhausted. Trips to restaurants, the mall, and even vacations may become impossible due to sensory issues or poor behavior. Large amounts of time and thousands of dollars are regularly spent going to doctors, speech therapists, occupational therapists, behavioral therapists and counselors. Schooling the child becomes a constant worry and battle. Is their child in the right educational setting and is the child getting the help he needs? Eventually children with autism become adults and then what happens to them? Most children with autism will forever be dependent on their parents and society.

While the family as a whole suffers, individuals and relationships in the family have unique challenges. The extra work of caring for a child with autism can stress parents. Research has shown the dramatic strain on marriage from caring for a child with autism.[8] These parents rarely have time for themselves individually, much less time for themselves as a couple. Another important area to consider is the toll on siblings. The parents are so busy taking care of the child with autism that the other children may not receive the time or resources they need. These parents are doing the best they can but are often pushed beyond their limits.

The financial impacts to society and families are severe. Schools are burdened with educating a growing population of special needs children. The lifetime societal cost for each child with autism is estimated at $3.2 million.[9] Because insurance companies consider autism to be a "psychological developmental disability" and not "medical," the treatment costs are not covered, leaving families to cover the costs. Intensive therapies such as speech, occupational, or behavioral can cost tens of thousands of dollars per year. Many families file for bankruptcy because of the financial burden.

What about the future of our society? We have a growing portion of our children who may never be able to fully function in school or in the workforce. They may never live independently and support themselves. They may never marry, have children, or have a job. While not all children with autism are so limited in their futures, many are, and the negative effects on society should not be underestimated.

The Solution

It is clear that we must curb this epidemic and help our children. The consequences of inaction are dire.

One solution would be to treat the growing number of children who have already acquired autism and ADHD. This is what I do in my medical practice. I treat hundreds of children with autism and ADHD. With my care and that of other therapists, many get better. They may no longer suffer from seizures, stomach pains, diarrhea, skin rashes, wheezing, mood swings, and anxiety. Some children improve so much that they no longer have an autism diagnosis.

Unfortunately, most children with autism still have major issues with learning and social interactions. How they will function as adults is of concern. Autism encompasses a large spectrum, with some children being so severely affected that they are unable to speak or interact with others. These children will need one-on-one personalized care every day for the rest of their lives. Often this will be from a parent. Other children may have speech delays and some repetitive rigid behavior—their outlook is obviously better but still uncertain. While we must strive to treat every child with autism, we need a better solution. A more effective solution would be to prevent autism and ADHD from occurring in the first place.

For the past 6 years, I have reviewed hundreds of published studies that examined multiple potential causes of autism and ADHD. I have researched many approaches that I and other doctors use to help these children get better and then applied this information to determine how these approaches could be used in prevention. From this research, it is clear to me that the solution for autism and ADHD is to help women understand and control their individual risk factors starting prior to pregnancy.

Autism is a biomedical (human biology and physiology) problem, which manifests significant physical and psychological symptoms. Children with autism often have digestive problems, seizures, poor muscle tone, growth issues, high toxin levels, and recurring chronic infections. It is time for the pediatric medical community to assert the medical basis for autism and to cease defining autism only by the psychological symptoms it produces. With a more accurate definition, we can examine the risk factors and implement prevention programs.

A good example of the kind of prevention program needed for autism is the public health effort that has been made to prevent cardiovascular (heart) disease. Even though more research needs to be done, the causes of heart disease are known through research to be multi-factorial. Rather than wait until more research is conducted, the medical community and policy makers have stepped up to the challenge of preventing heart disease. Doctors now advise their patients to reduce their risk for heart disease by eating a healthy diet, maintaining a healthy weight, getting exercise, and not smoking. Most people know that their risk for heart disease is the product of their family history, stress, and lifestyle.

Prevention programs for autism are not yet in place. Women are not aware that their family history and their health (especially before pregnancy) are related to their risk for autism. We need new policies, funding, clinical studies, and education directed at the prevention of autism. The prevention practices in this book are safe and contribute to an overall improvement in the health of the mother and baby. I describe approaches that are precautionary—approaches that lead to increased health *and* prevention of autism. Even though more research needs to be done, we know enough now to prevent the burden of autism.

CHAPTER 1 REFERENCES

1. Center for Disease Control and Prevention. Autism Spectrum Disorders prevalence studies of eight year olds - Autism and Developmental Disabilities Monitoring (ADDM) Network Data for 2000, 2002, 2004, 2006, 2008, DH327.

2. Blumberg SJ, Bramlett MD, Kogan MD, Schieve LA, Jones JR, Lu MC. Changes in Prevalence of parent-reported autism spectrum disorder in school-aged U.S. Children: 2007 to 2011–2012. *National Health Statistics Report.* 2013 Mar 20; 65. DH614.

3. Ibid.

4. Baird G, Simonoff E, Pickles A, Chandler S, Loucas T, Meldrum D, Charman T. Prevalence of disorders of the autism spectrum in a population cohort of children in South Thames: the Special Needs and Autism Project (SNAP). *Lancet.* 2006 Jul 15;368(9531):210-5. DH2.

5. Kim, YS. Et al. Prevalence of autism spectrum disorders in a total population sample. *Am Jour of Psychiatry.* 2011;168:904-912. DH4.

6. Centers for Disease Control and Prevention prevalence studies of eight year olds.

7. Boyle CA, Boulet S, Schieve LA, Cohen RA, Blumberg SJ, Yeargin-Allsopp M, Visser S, Kogan MD. Trends in the prevalence of developmental disabilities in US children, 1997-2008. *Pediatrics.* 2011 Jun;127(6):1034-42. DH3.

8. Hartley SL, Barker ET, Seltzer MM, Floyd F, Greenberg J, Orsmond G, Bolt D. The relative risk and timing of divorce in families of children with an autism spectrum disorder. *J Fam Psychol.* 2010 Aug;24(4):449-57. DH616.

9. Ganz ML. The lifetime distribution of the incremental societal costs of autism. *Arch Pediatric Adoles Med.* 2007 Apr;161(4):343-9. DH329. *Pediatric Adoles Med.* 2007 Apr;161(4):343-9. DH329.

2

Risk Factors

What causes autism and ADHD? This is the big question. From the 1990s, medical researchers have been studying and publishing papers on dozens of potential causes of autism and ADHD. Definitive causes have been elusive. The CDC states that "...there are likely many causes for multiple types of ASDs... including environmental, biologic and genetic factors."[1] Fortunately, researchers have identified many risk factors for autism.

This chapter will introduce these risk factors. Later chapters will provide the background and research studies to show their relation to autism and ADHD and methods for their control.

This chapter will also examine the role that genes and environment play in the causes of autism. Finally, we will examine an exciting new field that examines the interplay of genes and the environment, called *epigenetics*.

Risk Factors

We regularly see media reports of new risk factors for autism and ADHD. *Risk factors* refer to something in the medical history of a family member or the child that means the child is more likely to develop a disease. The risk factor does not mean that the child will definitely develop autism or ADHD. Usually the more risk factors, the more likely the child will acquire one of these diseases.

Fortunately, most of these risk factors are modifiable—meaning that the risk can be altered. Most risk factors are negative risk factors, meaning that their presence is related to a higher risk of autism and ADHD. Some risk factors are positive (or protective) meaning they are associated with less incidence of autism. By managing these risk factors, the chance of acquiring autism or ADHD will be reduced: the ultimate goal of autism and ADHD prevention.

Risk Factors Associated with Family History

When considering autism, the most important illnesses to identify in family members fall into two primary categories: developmental disorders and allergy/autoimmune diseases. The strongest association from family history is if a previous child has autism. In this case, the next child is at greatly increased risk.[2] If the mother or father has autism or ADHD, this also increases the risk.

In both allergies and autoimmune disease, the immune system isn't working properly. The immune system is designed to fight infections. If it detects something thought to be harmful to the body, it will react regardless if it is a true infection or not. For example, when people are exposed to pollen in the spring, those with allergies to pollen have an immune system that is fighting the pollen (even though the pollen is not an infection). This is where the sneezing and wheezing come from.

Autoimmune disease is when the immune system attacks otherwise healthy tissues. In autoimmune thyroid disease, the body attacks its own thyroid. In rheumatoid arthritis, the joints are targeted. When the immune system is activated, the result is inflammation. As an example, if you hit your hand it becomes swollen, red, warm, and tender—the hallmark signs of inflammation.

If there is a family history of allergies and autoimmune disease, especially in the mother, there is increased risk of the child developing autism.[3] It is unclear why there is this association. Both allergies and autoimmune disease are associated with an abnormal immune system reaction and inflammation. If the mother has this inflammation, there may be abnormal immune signals transferred to the infant in utero. Research shows that the mother's immune system detects the fetus as foreign and begins to form antibodies.[4] These antibodies can cause inflammation in the fetus. The association may also be an indication of a genetic tendency toward inflammation, where the child is more likely to have abnormal immune reactions.

Family-related risk factors for autism

- Relative with autism or ADHD
- Allergies
- Autoimmune diseases (autoimmune thyroid disease, rheumatoid arthritis, or inflammatory bowel disease)

I commonly find these and the following prenatal risk factors in the histories of children with autism or ADHD.

Prenatal Risk Factors

A review of 64 published epidemiological studies (research of the patterns and distribution of health issues) shows that the following prenatal (before birth) risk factors result in increased chances of having a child with autism:[5]

- Advanced maternal age
- Advanced paternal age
- Time when prenatal care began
- Bleeding during pregnancy (may be due to hypoxia)
- Gestational diabetes
- Maternal asthma
- Maternal allergies
- Stress during pregnancy
- Maternal use of medication during pregnancy (e.g. psychiatric)
- Urban location during pregnancy
- Increased pregnancy complications
- Maternal obesity

- Maternal smoking (ADHD specifically)
- Pesticide exposure
- Heavy metal exposure (e.g. lead or mercury)
- Gender of the child (boys have a greater risk than girls)

While researching this book I found many additional risk factors in the areas of nutrition, digestion, and toxins.

Causes: Genes or Environment

Initially, researchers argued as to whether genes or the environment caused autism. Unfortunately it is not that simple. Millions of dollars have been spent trying to find a genetic cause. Some genes have been found to be involved, but only in a few select children. Environmental factors have been discovered that increase risk in some children. Again, not one particular environmental factor is seen in all children.

Many researchers now consider the causes to be some interaction of genes with the environment.[6,7] There is not one gene that interacts with one environmental factor to cause autism. Autism is a spectrum of disorders with problems in speech, behavior, and social interactions that can be mild to severe. The accompanying problems such as seizures, allergies, infections, and digestive issues also vary from nonexistent to incapacitating.

In order to learn more about the genetic and environmental factors in autism, a long-term study was initiated in 2003 called the *CHARGE (Childhood Autism Risks from Genetics and the Environment)* study.[8] The study enrolled children from ages 2 to 5; some were diagnosed with autism, some with another type of developmental delay, and some with no developmental issues. Numerous research articles have been published from analysis of the data gained in this study. They found causative factors that span the range from specific genes to environmental exposures in the parents. We need to understand all of these factors, but most importantly, we need to know how these factors interact to produce the symptoms in these children.

Genes and Autism

Genes are our body's most basic biological building blocks. Genes hold the information to build and maintain an organism's cells and pass genetic traits to offspring. Research into the causes of autism initially concentrated on finding that one, single gene that would be the key to unlocking the cause of autism.

Genetic research has focused on finding a mutation or a change in the DNA (deoxyribonucleic acid). Research has found some changes in the DNA of genes on specific chromosomes associated with autism, such as numbers 2q, 7q, and 15q. Yet these account for very few children with autism. Often when the parents are tested, they have the same DNA changes yet do not have autism. Obviously something is affecting how those genes are functioning (called "expression") within a child with autism.

Several genetic syndromes have been discovered that are associated with autism. Many of these have been around a long time and children with these syndromes have always had problems. For example, Down syndrome is a genetic change with an extra copy of the 21st chromosome. Children with Down syndrome have always had developmental delays. Now many of them are also being diagnosed with autism. Overall genetic syndromes account for 5 to 10% of the autism cases.[9] If approximately 5% to 10% of cases have a genetic mutation, then the other 90% to 95% must have other factors involved.

Our ability to test genes has increased several hundredfold with microarray technology. We are able to discover more genes but the technology hasn't revealed the cause for the increase in these diseases.

Genetic syndromes associated with Autism (about 5-10% of total)

- Angelman's syndrome
- Tuberous sclerosis
- Fragile X syndrome
- Rett syndrome
- Phenylketonuria
- Joubert syndrome
- Mobius syndrome
- Other chromosomal disorders: chromosome 2q, 7q, and 15q
- Down syndrome
- Cohen syndrome
- Smith-Lemli-Opitz syndrome

Environmental Risk Factors

When people think about environmental causes of a disease, they usually think about something that a person is exposed to. This exposure changes how the body functions. An environmental factor can be something a person eats, drinks, breathes in, or touches. It can be a one-time occurrence or happen over a lifetime. With autism, we should be concerned about exposures that a future mother or father may have even before conception.

The question then becomes: how does something a person consumes, for instance pesticides on food, cause changes in the body that lead to health issues like autism? The substance must physically change function. We know that some substances cause damage to the DNA, which would lead to genetic change. Other substances can lead to a change in how the gene is controlled. Toxins in this category, called *carcinogens or mutagens,* affect the DNA and increase the risk of cancer. Cigarette smoke contains many toxins, and exposure over a lifetime is known to increase the risk of lung and other types of cancer. Damage to the DNA from a chemical when a child is in utero can lead to birth defects or miscarriage. These chemicals are called *teratogens.* Again, it seems the environment is affecting the DNA and making it difficult to separate the two.

We do know that some toxins damage the nervous system, especially a growing nervous system, which is why a baby in utero or a young child is vulnerable. These are called *neurotoxins.* We have known for decades that many of these toxins cause birth defects and neurological problems. Below is a list of some known neurotoxins.

Toxins associated with neurodevelopmental disabilities[10]

- Mercury
- Lead
- PCBs (polychlorinated biphenyl)
- Arsenic
- Manganese
- Organophosphate pesticides
- DDT (dichlorodiphenyltrichloroethane)
- ETOH (ethanol)

One of the primary difficulties with analyzing a woman's environmental toxin risk is that most toxic effects are cumulative over a lifetime. It is very difficult to measure how much a person has been exposed to. In addition, we are exposed to a multitude of different chemicals that can combine to produce negative effects. Combining chemicals can have synergistic effects, so they may be more harmful than a chemical alone. Chemicals are rarely tested in combination and their true adverse effects on human health are largely unknown.

In the U.S., a substance is deemed healthy unless proven otherwise. In Europe, a substance must be proven to be healthy before it can be used commercially. For a healthy baby, women should adopt the European model and only expose themselves to substances that they know to be safe.

Epigenetics

From the above information on genetic and environmental causes, it is clear that the cause of autism is not strictly genetic or environmental. Genes are affected by the environment. There is a constant interplay between the two that cannot be separated. This interrelationship is best defined by the term *epigenetics.*

Epigenetics is the biological response to an environmental stressor. From the beginning of conception, once we have our DNA or genetic material, our DNA doesn't change. What does change is the message to the DNA, whether it should turn on specific genes or not. Cellular material called the *epigenome* is adjacent to the gene, and our environment can influence the epigenome to change its message.

Figure 1 below depicts the function of the epigenome. Environmental stressors from the outside change the instructions that tell the DNA what to do.

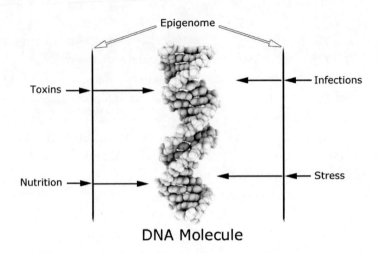

Figure 1 – Epigenome interface between DNA and environment

Environmental factors, such as diet (including prenatal diet), smoking, pesticides, stress, and even parent age can change the gene expression.[11] Research is beginning to focus on the epigenome for many chronic diseases including autism.[12,13] To me, this is where we need to focus our efforts in understanding causation.

One of the more frightening aspects of epigenetics is the effect from one generation to the next. A toxic exposure to the mother even before she is pregnant can change a message to the DNA. This altered message is then passed to her child during pregnancy and then potentially to her child's children or her grandchildren. Consider that when a female fetus is developing inside her mother, the fetus already has eggs in her growing ovary for reproduction of her own children. If a mother is exposed to a toxin, not only is her baby exposed to the toxin, but also her baby's eggs and therefore her potential grandchildren! When a woman is pregnant, any exposure she has affects not only her child but also the genetic material for her grandchild. This is called *transgenerational epigenetics*.

In order for the epigenome to change its instruction to the DNA, there has to be a chemical reaction at the molecular level. One of the chemical mechanisms that change the epigenome is a process called *methylation*.

In methylation, a chemical compound called a methyl group is added to an epigenome protein. This chemistry is important because the process of methylation is also the same type of chemistry that is weak in children with autism. Often methylation is also weak in their family members and this may manifest in other illnesses. Children with autism and their family members then have problems regulating the epigenome and therefore may be more at risk from toxins and poor diet. In addition, the process of methylation is critical for other pathways of detoxification in the body or the ability of the body to naturally remove toxins. This may lead to an even greater susceptibility to the harmful effects of toxins in those with autism.

From epigenetics arises hope. What gives us hope is that this methylation weakness is reversible. Healthy environmental factors can direct methylation to change the epigenome back to its original state. Animal studies have shown that giving pregnant mice additional B vitamins, which are critical for methylation, results in healthier offspring.[14,15] If it is possible to reverse epigenetic changes, then prevention becomes possible.

Summary

The argument as to whether autism is caused by either genetic or environmental risk factors needs to end. Our environment and our genes are intertwined in ways that are still too complex to dissect. Epigenetics weaves these two factors together by explaining how environmental risk factors influence the control of the genes. In-depth research into the epigenetic causation of autism and ADHD needs to continue and accelerate.

Dozens of published medical research studies show us that there are numerous risk factors for autism before, during and after pregnancy. We must act now to help mothers identify, manage, and reduce (when possible) their risk factors before, during and after pregnancy. When risk factors are reduced, we will reduce our rates of autism and ADHD, which is the ultimate goal of prevention.

CHAPTER 2 REFERENCES

1. CDC autism facts website accessed May 4, 2013.

2. Constantino JN, Zhang Y, Frazier T, Abbacchi AM, Law P. Sibling recurrence and the genetic epidemiology of autism. *Am J Psychiatry.* 2010 November;167(11):1349-1356. DH143.

3. Atladottir HO, et al. Association of family history of autoimmune diseases and autism spectrum disorders. *Pediatrics.* 2009 Aug;124(2):687-94. DH145.

4. Fox E, Amaral D, Van de Water J. Maternal and fetal antibrain antibodies in development and disease. *Dev Neurobiol.* 2012 Oct;72(10):1327-34. DH408.

5. Gardener H, Spiegelman D, Buka SL. Prenatal risk factors for autism: comprehensive meta-analysis. *Br J Psychiatry.* 2009 Jul;195(1):7-14. DH387.

6. Hertz-Picciotto I, Croen LA, Hansen R, Jones CR, van de Water J, Pessah IN. The CHARGE study: an epidemiologic investigation of genetic and environmental factors contributing to autism. *Environ Health Perspect.* 2006 Jul;114(7):1119-25. DH385.

7. Landrigan PJ. What causes autism? Exploring the environmental contribution. *Curr Opin Pediatr.* 2010 Apr;22(2):219-25. DH264.

8. Hert-Picciotto 2006.

9. Landrigan 2010.

10. Landrigan 2010.

11. Herbert MR, Russo JP, Yang S, Roohi J, Mlaxill M, Kahler SG, Cremer L, Hatchwell E. Autism and environmental genomics. *J Neuro Toxicology.* 2006;27(5):671-84. DH349.

12. Schanen NC. Epigenetics of autism spectrum disorders. *Hum Mol Genet.* 2006;15 Spec No 2:R138-150. DH137.

13. Waterland RA, Jirtle RI. Transposable elements: targets for early nutritional effects on epigenetic gene regulation. *Mol Cell Biol* 2003;23:5293-300. DH350.

14. Chan J, Deng L, Mikael LG, Yan J, Pickell L, Wu Q, Caudill MA, Rozen R. Low dietary choline and low dietary riboflavin during pregnancy influence reproductive outcomes and heart development in mice. *Am J Clin Nutr.* 2010 Apr;91(4):1035-43. DH567.

15. Waterland RA, Dolinoy DC, Lin JR, Smith CA, Shi X, Tahiliani KG. Maternal methyl supplements increase offspring DNA methylation at Axin Fused. *Genesis.* 2006 Sep;44(9):401-6. DH407.

3

The Power of Prevention

The next step in developing a comprehensive autism and ADHD prevention program came from comparing the many risk factors for autism with my own clinical experience treating children with these diseases.

The Triangle of Prevention

Further clues for prevention strategies came from how I treat hundreds of children with autism and ADHD. I realized that I focused primarily on three areas: (1) healthy diet/nutrition, (2) strong digestion, and (3) detoxification. If these three areas are the cornerstones of successful treatment, then they must be important in prevention. If I could explain to parents why we need to treat each of these areas when their child has autism, then I could explain to potential parents, pregnant women, and mothers of young children why we need to address each of these areas to prevent autism.

In order to simplify the understanding of the prevention program, I developed the *Triangle of Prevention* and it focuses on these three areas. Each area is important individually, but also in relation to each other.

1. Healthy diet/nutrition (essential nutrition, critical supplementation, and harmful food avoidance)
2. Strong digestion (probiotics, absorption, and elimination)
3. Detoxification (avoiding/removing toxins and improving the body's detoxification system)

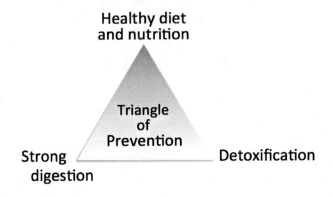

Figure 2 – Triangle of Prevention

Hypothesis

I reviewed the published medical studies for one risk factor for each of these three areas. If my clinical autism treatment approach, which reduces the symptoms of autism, aligns closely with these risk factor studies, then there is strong justification that helping mothers to address the modifiable risk factors will prevent many cases of autism.

Autism Prevention Hypothesis

(1) Children with autism present with a variety of negative symptoms. We have effective treatments for these symptoms.

(2) We know that there are dozens of risk factors for autism, many of them modifiable.

By reducing risk factors starting before pregnancy, we can prevent symptoms of autism from occurring in new children and we will reduce the incidence of autism.

To test this hypothesis, I examined evidenced-based research studies to see if there was scientific support for the Triangle of Prevention. I examined one risk factor in each of the three areas: nutrition, digestion, and detoxification.

Hypothesis Test for Nutrition – Risk Factor: Omega-3 Fatty Acids

Most people know omega-3 fatty acids such as fish oil or cod liver oil. When I began practicing integrative medicine and later working on this prevention book, my father responded to me, "You mean we are back to cod liver oil?" Yes, we are! Most people now know about the many health benefits of taking cod liver oil or omega-3 fats. Many obstetricians recommend pregnant woman take omega-3 fatty acid supplements.

My hypothesis test for nutrition begins with the concept that if something important is missing before and/or during pregnancy, it will have a negative effect on the future development of the child. For this example, studies show that an insufficient amount of omega-3 fatty acids consumed during pregnancy leads to infant developmental delays in social behavior, speech, and cognition, see Figure 3. Scientific studies referenced shown in the figure lend strong support for the hypothesis that adequate levels of omega-3 fatty acids in mothers and babies will lead to children with better neurologic development and decreased autistic symptoms. These studies show that children with autism, who have delays in social behavior, speech, and cognition, also have fatty

21

acid deficiencies. However, symptoms of autism decrease following omega-3 supplementation.

New research supports the hypothesis. A 2013 study found that women supplemented with omega-3 fatty acids during and after pregnancy had more normal size babies at birth and was associated with better growth during infancy.[1] A 2012 study found that maternal omega-3 supplementation was associated with better cognitive skills in young children.[2]

Therefore, it makes sense that if women and new babies get adequate levels of omega-3 fatty acids, their risk for autism will be reduced.

Omega-3 Fatty Acids and Autism Hypothesis

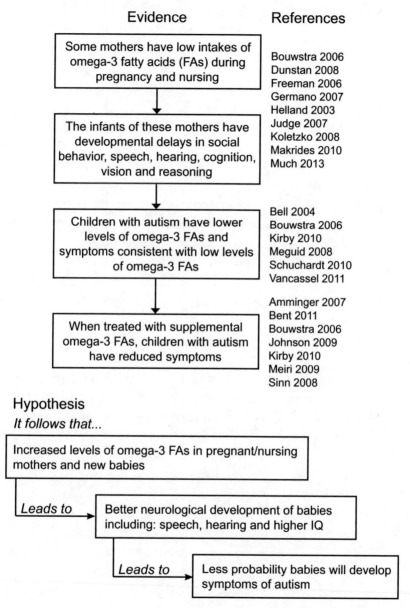

Evidence

References

Some mothers have low intakes of omega-3 fatty acids (FAs) during pregnancy and nursing

Bouwstra 2006
Dunstan 2008
Freeman 2006
Germano 2007
Helland 2003
Judge 2007
Koletzko 2008
Makrides 2010
Much 2013

The infants of these mothers have developmental delays in social behavior, speech, hearing, cognition, vision and reasoning

Children with autism have lower levels of omega-3 FAs and symptoms consistent with low levels of omega-3 FAs

Bell 2004
Bouwstra 2006
Kirby 2010
Meguid 2008
Schuchardt 2010
Vancassel 2011

When treated with supplemental omega-3 FAs, children with autism have reduced symptoms

Amminger 2007
Bent 2011
Bouwstra 2006
Johnson 2009
Kirby 2010
Meiri 2009
Sinn 2008

Hypothesis

It follows that...

Increased levels of omega-3 FAs in pregnant/nursing mothers and new babies

Leads to → Better neurological development of babies including: speech, hearing and higher IQ

Leads to → Less probability babies will develop symptoms of autism

Figure 3 - Omega-3 Fatty Acids and Autism Hypothesis

Hypothesis Test for Digestion – Risk Factor: Probiotic Bacteria

Probiotics are the "good bacteria" in our intestines and are essential to our digestive health. Probiotics are important not only for digestive function but also for the immune system. In fact, approximately 70% of our immune system is in the intestine. These good bacteria also happen to exist in the genital tract of women.

Infants primarily get probiotics from the mother during a vaginal birth as the baby ingests probiotics by passing through the birth canal.[3] Infants may also receive probiotics from breastfeeding. A cesarean or C-section birth does not allow infants to obtain probiotics from the mother, and bottle-feeding does not provide probiotics. If the mother does not have an adequate supply of probiotics, then she cannot pass them onto her infant, even during a vaginal delivery and nursing.

Why would a mother not have an adequate level of probiotics? Antibiotic use (often overuse) is the most common reason probiotics are destroyed. Antibiotics are readily given for infections, and they are also added to our food supply and vaccines. It is no wonder that many women have low levels of these important probiotics. Antibiotic use in infants can also lead to destruction of good bacteria.

Inadequate probiotics in babies leads to many digestive symptoms such as colic, gastroesophageal reflux, food allergies, and feeding issues. Many of these symptoms are more commonly seen after C-section births. Interestingly, more children with autism and ADHD are born by C-section than children without these disorders.

Although almost all children have occasional digestive problems, a higher proportion of children with autism—in fact, 70%—suffer from these issues.[4] Digestive problems often involve food allergies/sensitivities and infections in the intestines, which can affect behavior. *The Gut and Psychology Syndrome*, a book by Dr. Natasha Campbell-McBride, illustrates the interrelationship between the brain, behavior, and the digestive system. One cornerstone to treating children with autism is to address their digestive disorders.

The hypothesis test for digestion (Figure 4) shows that supplementing probiotics in mothers-to-be leads to less digestive problems in infants, which subsequently leads to less behavioral issues frequently seen in children with autism. Treating digestion problems of children with autism reduces behavioral problems. Therefore, it makes sense that ensuring mothers and babies have adequate probiotic bacteria will reduce their chances for digestive problems—a common symptom of children with autism.

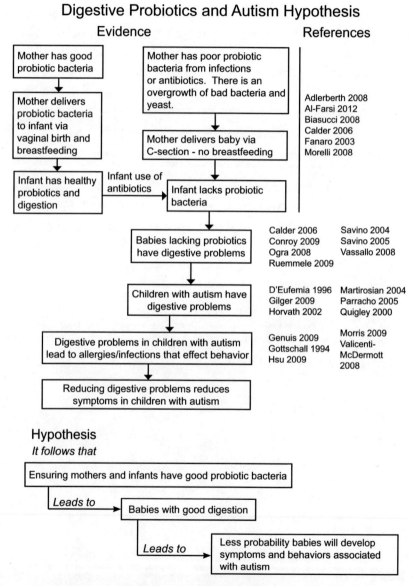

Figure 4 – Digestive Probiotics and Autism Hypothesis

Hypothesis Test for Toxins—Risk Factor: Mercury and Lead

The diet and digestion examples described earlier are concerned about the lack of something critical. However, this hypothesis test for toxins is concerned about the addition of something harmful. Research shows that if mothers are exposed to mercury and/or lead when they are pregnant, their infants show specific developmental delays. These delays include problems with attention, which is seen in most children with autism and all children with ADHD. Other delays include those of language and the sensory processing system such as vision and hearing. Both mercury and lead are potent neurotoxins. In plain terms, they poison the nervous system, and a developing nervous system is particularly vulnerable to harm.

Many children with autism have elevated levels of heavy metals (Figure 5). They also exhibit symptoms consistent with neurologic problems that are seen with mercury and lead exposure. During treatment, as mercury and lead are slowly removed, these children get better, and their language and cognition improve. Therefore, preventing exposure to these metals (as much as possible) will lower the levels of these toxins in children and subsequently result in less neurologic and developmental issues including autism.

Toxin testing, measurement, and removal are complex. In my opinion we need to focus a lot of new research in this area—for our children and our future children.

Toxins Mercury/Lead and Autism Hypothesis

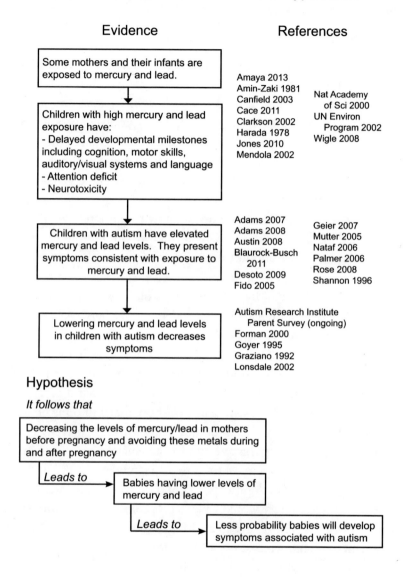

Evidence   References

Some mothers and their infants are exposed to mercury and lead.

Amaya 2013
Amin-Zaki 1981
Canfield 2003 — Nat Academy of Sci 2000
Cace 2011 — UN Environ Program 2002
Clarkson 2002
Harada 1978 — Wigle 2008
Jones 2010
Mendola 2002

Children with high mercury and lead exposure have:
- Delayed developmental milestones including cognition, motor skills, auditory/visual systems and language
- Attention deficit
- Neurotoxicity

Children with autism have elevated mercury and lead levels. They present symptoms consistent with exposure to mercury and lead.

Adams 2007
Adams 2008 — Geier 2007
Austin 2008 — Mutter 2005
Blaurock-Busch 2011 — Nataf 2006
Desoto 2009 — Palmer 2006
Fido 2005 — Rose 2008
Shannon 1996

Lowering mercury and lead levels in children with autism decreases symptoms

Autism Research Institute Parent Survey (ongoing)
Forman 2000
Goyer 1995
Graziano 1992
Lonsdale 2002

Hypothesis

It follows that

Decreasing the levels of mercury/lead in mothers before pregnancy and avoiding these metals during and after pregnancy

Leads to

Babies having lower levels of mercury and lead

Leads to

Less probability babies will develop symptoms associated with autism

Figure 5 – Toxins Mercury/Lead and Autism Hypothesis

These hypothesis diagrams show that we can reduce the incidence of autism through modification of risk factors. While these hypothesis diagrams only show three risk factors, the remaining chapters of the book will show dozens of risk factors that also can be modified to prevent autism and ADHD.

Challenges of Researching a Prevention Program

In an ideal world, we would be able to confirm a prevention program by doing clinical studies. The type of study that is considered the gold standard is the *randomized double blind placebo controlled trial.* That string of words means that we take two groups of people to study, for example, two groups of women who are pregnant. Then we randomly assign one group of women to receive one treatment and the other to receive no treatment. As an example, we could give one group omega-3 fatty acids from fish oil and the other group will receive no fish oil. We don't want one group to know they are receiving the good oils and the other are not receiving any so we would need to give a fish flavored oil to the group not receiving the fish oil. Then we follow the pregnant women through the end of their pregnancies and then follow the health of their children. At two years old, we would then see how many of these children had autism if their mothers received fish oil versus those whose mothers did not receive fish oil. If the fish oil helped prevent autism, there should be fewer children with autism from the mothers who took fish oil during pregnancy. Now here is the serious ethical problem from doing a randomized double blind placebo controlled trial for prevention: we already know that fish oil is helpful for brain development, so we cannot do a study where we prevent a woman from taking something that we know is beneficial.

Alternatively, suppose we want to do a study on the negative effects of mercury on the development of a child. In order to perform the gold standard in research we would have to give some pregnant women mercury and others would have to avoid it. It would be unethical to give a pregnant woman mercury, not to mention no pregnant woman would volunteer to take a known neurotoxin!

To confirm or deny the entire prevention program, we would do these studies for each of the known risk factors. However, each study would have serious ethical issues because we cannot keep from women approaches that we know would help baby health or give them substances that we know harm baby's health.

Summary

Because we cannot ethically do these gold standard research studies to validate an autism and ADHD prevention program, we need to take what we do know about biochemistry, risk factors and risk factor modification, and implement the program now. We already do this for other health concerns, such as heart disease.

The many evidence-based studies on risk factors strongly indicate that the prevention program described in this book will be successful. While this program is aimed at having children free of autism and ADHD, it will also improve the overall health of both the mother and the child. Our children's health is at stake. We must act now to save our children.

CHAPTER 3 REFERENCES

1. Much D, Brunner S, Vollhardt C, Schmid D, Sedlmeier EM, Brüderl M, Heimberg E, Bartke N, Boehm G, Bader BL, Amann-Gassner U, Hauner H. Effect of dietary intervention to reduce the n-6/n-3 fatty acid ratio on maternal and fetal fatty acid profile and its relation to offspring growth and body composition at 1 year of age. *Eur J Clin Nutr.* 2013 Jan 23. DH570.

2. Larqué E, Gil-Sánchez A, Prieto-Sánchez MT, Koletzko B. Omega 3 fatty acids, gestation and pregnancy outcomes. *Br J Nutr.* 2012 Jun;107 Suppl 2:S77-84. DH571.

3. Penders J, et al. Factors influencing the composition of the intestinal microbiota in early infancy. *Pediatrics.* 2006;118(2):511-512. DH78.

4. Buie T, et al. Evaluation, diagnosis and treatment of gastrointestinal disorders in individuals with ASDs: a consensus report. *Pediatrics.* 2010;125(suppl 1):S1-S18. DH56.

Omega-3 Fatty Acids and Autism Hypothesis Diagram

Amminger GP, Berger GE, Schafer MR, Llier C, Friedrich MH, Feucht M. Omega-3 fatty acids supplementation in children with autism double-blind randomized, placebo-controlled pilot study. *Biol Psychiatry.* 2007;61(4):551-553. DH28.

Bell JG, MacKinlay EE, Dick JR, MacDonald DJ, Boyle RM, Glen AC. Essential fatty acids and phospholipase A2 in autistic spectrum disorders. *Prostaglandins Leukot Essent Fatty Acids.* 2004;71(4):201-204. DH29.

Bent S, Bertoglio K, Ashwood P, Bostrom A, Hendren RL. A pilot randomized controlled trial of omega-3-fatty acids for autism spectrum disorder. *J Autism Dev Disord.* 2011 May;41(5):545-54. DH30.

Bouwstra H, Dijck-Brouwer J, Decsi T, Boehm G, Boersma ER, Muskiet FA, Hadders-Algra M. Neurologic condition of healthy term infants at 18 months: positive association with venous umbilical DHA status and negative association with umbilical trans-fatty acids. *Pediatr Res.* 2006;60(3):334-339. DH31.

Dunstan JF, Simmer K, Dixon G, and Prescott SL. Cognitive assessment of children at age 2 ½ years after maternal fish oil supplementation in pregnancy: a randomized controlled trial. *Arch Dis Child Fetal Neonatal Ed.* 2008;93:F45-F50. DH32.

Freeman MP, Hibbeln JR, Wisner KL, Davis JM, Mischoulon D, Peet M, Keck PE Jr, Marangell LB, Richardson AJ, Lake J, Stoll AL. Omega-3 fatty acids: evidence basis for treatment and future research in psychiatry. *J Clin Psychiatry.* 2006;67;1954-1967. DH33.

Germano M. Plasma, red blood cells phospholipids and clinical evaluation after long chain omega-3 supplementation in children with attention deficit hyperactivity disorder (ADHD). *Nutr Neurosci.* 2007;10(1-2):1-9. DH34.

Helland IB, Smith L, Saarem K, Saugstad OD, Drevon CA. Maternal supplementation with very-long-chain n-3 fatty acids during pregnancy and lactation augments children's IQ at 4 years of age. *Pediatrics.* 2003;11(1):e39-e44. DH35.

Johnson M, Ostlund S, Fransson G, Kadesjo B, Gillberg C. Omega-3/omega-6 fatty acids for attention deficit hyperactivity disorder: a randomized placebo-controlled trial in children and adolescents. *J Atten Disord.* 2009;12(5):394-401. DH39.

Judge MP, Harel O, Lammi-Keefe C. Maternal consumption of a docosahexaenoic acid-containing functional food during pregnancy: benefit for infant performance on problem-solving but not on recognition memory tasks at age 9 mo. *Am J Clin Nutr.* 2007;85(6):1572-1577. DH40.

Kirby A, Woodward A, Jackson S, Wang Y, Crawford MA. Childrens' learning and behavior and the association with cheek cell polyunsaturated fatty acid levels. *Res Dev Disabil.* 2010;31(3):731-742. DH41.

Koletzko B, Lien E, Agostoni C, Böhles H, Campoy C, Cetin I, Decsi T, Dudenhausen JW, Dupont C, Forsyth S, Hoesli I, Holzgreve W, Lapillonne A, Putet G, Secher NJ, Symonds M, Szajewska H, Willatts P, Uauy R; World Association of Perinatal Medicine Dietary Guidelines Working Group. The roles of long-chain polyunsaturated fatty acids in pregnancy, lactation and infancy: review of current knowledge and consensus recommendations. *J Perinat Med.* 2008;36(1):5-14. DH42.

Makrides M, Gibson RA, McPhee AJ, Yelland L, Quinlivan J, Ryan P; DOMInO Investigative Team. Effect of DHA supplementation during pregnancy on maternal depression and neurodevelopment of young children: a randomized controlled trial. *JAMA.* 2010;304(15):1675-1683. DH43.

Meguid NA, Atta H, Gouda A, Khalil R. Role of polyunsaturated fatty acids in the management of Egyptian children with autism. *Clin Biochem.* 2008;41:1044-1048. DH44.

Meiri G, Bichovsky Y, Belmaker RH. Omega 3 fatty acid treatment in autism. *J Child Adolesc Psychopharmacol.* 2009;19(4):449-451. DH45.

Much D, Brunner S, Vollhardt C, Schmid D, Sedlmeier EM, Brüderl M, Heimberg E, Bartke N, Boehm G, Bader BL, Amann-Gassner U, Hauner H. Effect of dietary intervention to reduce the n-6/n-3 fatty acid ratio on maternal and fetal fatty acid profile and its relation to offspring growth and body composition at 1 year of age. *Eur J Clin Nutr.* 2013 Jan 23. DH570.

Schuchardt JP, Huss M, Stauss-Grabo M, Hahn A. Significance of long-chain polyunsaturated fatty acids (PUFAs) for the development and behaviour of children. *Eur J Pediatr.* 2010;169(2):149-164. DH46.

Sinn N. Nutritional and dietary influences on attention deficit hyperactivity disorder. *Nutr Rev.* 2008;66(10):558-568. DH47.

Vancassel S, Durand G, Barthélémy C, Lejeune B, Martineau J, Guilloteau D, Andrès C, Chalon S. Plasma fatty acid levels in autistic children. *Prostaglandins Leukot Essent Fatty Acids.* 2001;65(1):1-7. DH48.

Digestive Probiotics and Autism Hypothesis Diagram

Alderberth I. Factors influencing the establishment of the intestinal microbiota in infancy. *Nestle Nutr Workshop Ser Pediatr Program.* 2008;62:13-33. DH50.

Al-Farsi YM, Al-Sharbati MM, Waly MI, Al-Farsi OA, Al-Shafaee MA, Al-Khaduri MM, Trivedi MS, Deth RC. Effect of suboptimal breast-feeding on occurrence of autism: a case-control study. *Nutrition.* 2012 Jul;28(7-8):e27-32. DH558.

Biasucci G, Benenati B, Morelli L, Bessi E, Boehm G. Cesarean delivery may affect the early biodiversity of intestinal bacteria. *J Nutr.* 2008;138(9):1796S-1800S. DH55.

Calder PC, Krauss-Etschmann S, de Jong EC, Dupont C, Frick JS, Frokiaer H, Heinrich J, Garn H, Koletzko S, Lack G, Mattelio G, Renz H, Sangild PT, Schrezenmeir J, Stulnig TM, Thymann T, Wold AE, Koletzko B. Early nutrition and immunity – progress and perspectives. *Br J Nutr.* 2006;96(4):774-790. DH57.

Conroy ME, Shi HN, Walker WA. The long-term health effects of neonatal microbial flora. *Curr Opin Allergy Clin Immunol.* 2009;9(3):197-201. DH58.

D'Eufemia P, et al. Abnormal intestinal permeability in children with autism. *Acta Paediatr.* 1996;85(9):1076-1079. DH59.

Fanaro S, Chierici R, Guerrini P, Vigi V. Intestinal microflora in early infancy: composition and development. *Acta Paediatr Suppl.* 2003;91(441):48-55. DH95.

Genuis SJ, Bouchard TP. Celiac disease presenting as autism. *J Child Neurol.* 2009;25(1):114-119. DH62.

Gilger MA, Redel CA. Autism and the gut. *Pediatrics.* 2009;124(2):796-798. DH63.

Gottschell Elaine G. *Breaking the Vicious Cycle: Intestinal Health Through Diet.* Ontario: Kirkton Press. 1994.

Horvath K, Perman JA. Autism and gastrointestinal symptoms. *Curr Gastroenterol Rep.* 2002;4(3):251-258. DH68.

Hsu CL, Lin CY, Chen CL, Wang CM, Wong MK. The effects of a gluten and casein-free diet in children with autism: a case report. *Chang Gung Med J.* 2009;32(4):459-465. DH70.

Martirosian G. Anaerobic intestinal microflora in pathogenesis of autism. *Postepy Hig Med Dosw* (online) [in Polish]. 2004;58:349-351. DH71.

Morelli L. Postnatal development of intestinal microflora as influenced by infant nutrition. *J Nutr.* 2008;138(9):1791S-1795S. DH73.

Morris CR, Agin MC. Syndrome of allergy, apraxia, and malabsorption: characterization of a neurodevelopmental phenotype that responds to omega 3 and vitamin E supplementation. *Altern Ther Health Med.* 2009;15(4):34-43. DH74.

Ogra PL, Welliver RC Sr. Effects of early environment on mucosal immunologic homeostasis, subsequent immune responses and disease outcome. *Nestle Nutr Workshop Ser Pediatr Program.* 2008;61:145-181. DH76.

Parracho HM, Bingham MO, Gibson GR, McCartney AL. Differences between the gut microflora of children with autistic spectrum disorders and that of healthy children. *J Med Microbiol.* 2005;54(pt 10):987-991. DH77.

Penders J, et al. Factors influencing the composition of the intestinal microbiota in early infancy. *Pediatrics.* 2006;118(2):511-512. DH78.

Quigley EM, Hurley D. Autism and the gastrointestinal tract. *Am J Gastroenterol.* 2000;95(9):2154-2156. DH70.

Ruemmele FM, Bier D, Marteau P, Rechkemmer G, Bourdet-Sicard R, Walker WA, Goulet O. Clinical evidence for immunomodulatory effects of probiotic bacteria. *J Pediatr Gastroenterology Nutr.* 2009;48(2):126-141. DH80.

Savino F, Cresi F, Pautasso S, Palumeri E, Tullio V, Roana J, Silvestro L, Oggero R. Intestinal microflora in breastfed colicky and non-colicky infants. *Acta Paediatr.* 2004;93(6):825-829. DH81.

Savino F, Bailo E, Oggero R, Tullio V, Roana J, Carlone N, Cuffini AM, Silvestro L. Bacterial counts of intestinal Lactobacillus species in infants with colic. *Pediatr Allergy Immunol.* 2005 Feb;16(1):72-5. DH82.

Valinenti-McDermott M, McVicar K, Cohen HJ, Wershil BK, Shinnar S. Gastrointestinal symptoms in children with an autism spectrum disorder and language regression. *Pediatr Neurol.* 2008;39(6):392-398. DH86.

Vassallo MF, Walker WA. Neonatal microbial flora and disease outcome. *Nestle Nutr Workshop Ser Pediatr Program.* 2008;61:211-24. DH88.

Toxins Mercury/Lead and Autism Hypothesis Diagram

Adams JB, Romdalvik J, Ramanujam, VM, Legator MS. Mercury, lead and zinc in baby teeth of children with autism versus controls. *J Toxicol Environ Health.* 2007;70(12):1046-1051. DH278.

Adams JB, Romdalvik J, Livine KE, Hu LW. Mercury in first-cut baby hair of children with autism versus typically developing children. *Toxicol Environ Chem.* 2008;1-14, iFirst. DH279.

Amaya E, Gil F, Freire C, Olmedo P, Fernández-Rodríguez M, Fernández MF, Olea N. Placental concentrations of heavy metals in a mother-child cohort. *Environ Res.* 2013 Jan;120:63-70. DH515.

Amin-Zaki L, Majeed MA, Greenwood MR, Elhassani SB, Clarkson TW, Doherty RA. Methylmercury poisoning in the Iraqi suckling infant: a longitudinal study over five years. *J Appl Toxicol.* 1981;1:210-214. DH280.

Austin D. An epidemiological analysis of the 'autism as mercury poisoning' hypothesis. *In J Risk Saf Med.* 2008;20:135-142. DH281.

Autism Research Istitute. Parent Survey (ongoing). ARI: San Diego, CA, 2011. DH282.

Blaurock-Busch E, Amin OR, Rabah T. Heavy metals and trace elements in hair and urine of a sample of Arab children with autistic spectrum disorder. *Maedica (Buchar).* 2011 Oct;6(4):247-57. DH569.

Cace IB, Milardovic A, Prpic I, Krajina R, Petrovic O, Vukelic P, Spiric Z, Horvat M, Mazej D, Snoj J. Relationship between the prenatal exposure to low-level of mercury and the size of a newborn's cerebellum. *Med Hypotheses.* 2011;76(4):514-516. DH283.

Canfield RL, Henderson CR Jr, Cory-Slechta DA, Cox C, Jusko TA, Lanphear BP. Intellectual impairment in children with blood lead concentrations below 10 microg per deciliter. *N Engl J Med.* 2003;348:1517-1526. DH284.

Clarkson TW. The three modern faces of mercury. *Environ Health Perspect.* 2002;110(suppl 1):11-23. DH287.

DeSoto M. Ockham's razor and autism: The case for developmental neurotoxins contributing to a disease of neurodevelopment. *Neurotoxicogy.* 2009;30:331-337. DH248.

Fido A, Al-Saad S. Toxic trace elements in the hair of children with autism. *Autism.* 2005;9(3):290-298. DH290.

Forman J, Moline J, Cernichiari E, Sayegh S, Torres JC, Landrigan MM, Hudson J, Adel HN, Landrigan PJ. A cluster of pediatric metallic mercury exposure cases treated with meso-2,3-dimercaptosuccinic acid (DMSA). *Environ Health Perspect.* 2000;108(6):575-577. DH291.

Geier DA, Geier MR. A prospective study of mercury toxicity biomarkers in autistic spectrum disorders. *J Tox Env Health.* Part A, 2007;70:1723-1730. DH202.

Goyer RA, Cherian MC, Jones MM, Reigart JR. Role of chelating agents for prevention, intervention, and treatment of exposures to toxic metals. *Environ Health Perspect.* 1995;103(11):1048-1052. DH293.

Graziano JH, Lolacono NJ, Moulton T, Mitchell ME, Slavkovich V, Zarate C. Controlled study of meso-2,3-dimercaptosuccinic acid for the management of childhood lead intoxication. *J Pediatr.* 1992;120(1):133-139. DH294.

Jones L, Parker JD, Mendola P. Blood lead and mercury levels in pregnant women in the United States, 2003-2008. *NCHS Data Brief.* 2010;(52):1-8. DH283.

Lonsdale D, Shamberger RJ, Audhya T. Treatment of autism spectrum children with thiamine tetrahydrofurfuryl disulfide: a pilot study. *Neuroendocrinol Lett.* 2002;23(4):303-308. DH299.

Mendola P, Selevan SG, Gutter S, Rice D. Environmental factors associated with a spectrum of neurodevelopmental deficits. *Ment Retard Dev Diabil Res Rev.* 2002;8(3):188-197.

Mutter J, Naumann J, Schneider R, Walach H, Haley B. Mercury and autism: accelerating evidence? *Neuro Endocrinol Lett.* 2005;26(5):439-446. DH132.

Nataf R, Skorupka C, Amet L, Lam A, Springbett A, Lathe R. Porphyrinuria in childhood autistic disorder: implications for environmental toxicity. *Toxicol Appl Pharmacol.* 2006;214(2):99-108. DH302.

National Academy of Sciences. Toxicological effects of methylmercury. 2000. Key findings. http://dels.nas.edu/Report/Toxicological-Effects-Methylmercury/9899. Accessed January 2011. DH303.

Palmer RF, Blanchard S, Stein Z, Mandell D, Miller C. Environmental mercury release, special education rates, and autism disorder: an ecological study of Texas. *Health Place.* 2006;12(2):203-209. DH304.

Rose S, Melnyk S, Savenka A, Hubanks A, Jernigan S, Cleves M, James SL. The frequency of polymorphisms affecting lead and mercury toxicity among children with autism. *Am J Biochem Biotechnol.* 2008;4(2):85-94. DH306.

Shannon M, Graef JW. Lead intoxication in children with pervasive developmental disorders. *J Toxicol Clin Toxicol.* 1996;34(2):177-181. DH307.

United Nations Environment Programme. Chemicals: Mercury Programme. Global Mercury Assessment Report and Appendix. 2002. http://www.chem.unep.ch/mercury/report/final-report-download.htm. Accessed January 2011. DH308.

Wigle DT, Arbuckle TE, Turner MC, Berube A, Yang Q, Liu S, Krewski D. Epidemiologic evidence of relationships between reproductive and child health outcomes and environmental chemical contaminants. *J Toxicol Environ Health.* 2008;11(5-6):373-517. DH141.

Part 2

Before Pregnancy
Autism & ADHD Prevention

4

The Critical Time Before Pregnancy

Our health care system has a significant missing component: preconception care. How can women have healthy babies if they are not optimally healthy before they become pregnant? I believe that the health of a woman before pregnancy is the most important factor in having a child free of autism and ADHD.

Preparation for Pregnancy

The majority of women think about the health of the baby only once they are already pregnant. They don't think that anything they have done up to that point makes a difference in their baby's health. Only when pregnant do most women consider improving their diet, taking prenatal vitamins, and avoiding alcohol and cigarettes. However, most women don't know they are pregnant until well into the first trimester. By that time, the majority of the organs in the embryo are formed, and nutrition and toxins have already had an impact.

For example, research shows the importance of taking the vitamins folic acid[1] and vitamin B12[2] when a woman is pregnant. These vitamins are crucial to help prevent *neural tube defects*, which are defects in the formation of the spinal cord. Since the spinal cord is formed early in pregnancy, the folic acid can only be maximally effective if it is taken from the point before conception.

The Mother/Baby Health Connection

The health of the mother and baby are closely intertwined. This is obvious during pregnancy when the fetus is entirely dependent on the mother. However, the state of the mother's health before pregnancy also determines what she will provide for the child during pregnancy. Following pregnancy, nursing continues the bond. The mother determines the child's nutrition (positively or negatively) and we know that children with autism have nutritional deficiencies.[3] The mother also determines all the environmental factors the child will be exposed to.

This complex, multi-factorial mother/baby health connection makes it difficult for researchers to perform studies and to isolate true causes of health issues like autism. It is the premise of this book that the health of the mother and baby are intertwined and that the baby's health is vulnerable to conditions in the mother that often cause her no symptoms. The healthiest child will result from the healthiest mother before, during, and after pregnancy.

Health Improvement Before Pregnancy

The ideal time to start to use the Triangle of Prevention is before pregnancy. The prevention plan needs to include making changes in the three areas of diet, digestion, and toxins.

Diet and nutrition

It is important to begin with improving diet and nutrition. If a woman is well nourished before conception, she has the nutrition stores to support optimal growth of the child during pregnancy. Developing healthy eating habits takes time and education. Not everyone knows about the importance of organic foods but the health benefits are significant. A nutritious diet leads to a healthy weight, which will help improve fertility and lessen complications during pregnancy and delivery.

40

Digestion

The next step is to improve digestion. Healthy food only helps strengthen the body when it is properly digested and absorbed. Part of developing healthy digestion is having a balance of good bacteria in the intestine. We are only beginning to understand the profound effects these good bacteria have on the development of a baby's immune and digestive systems. Since a woman needs to pass these good bacteria to her infant, she is a vital link to her infant having a strong immune system.

Toxins

One of the most important aspects of the preconception period is that it is the only time that is safe for detoxification. Detoxifying is helping the body to remove toxins. As a person removes toxins from their body, these toxins pass through the blood, digestive system, and kidneys. In a pregnant woman, any chemical that passes through her blood stream will pass through the placenta and will be exposed to her baby. Since a fetus is extremely small and is in the process of growing and developing, any chemical exposure can have a profound negative impact. Similarly, a nursing mother should not detoxify during breast-feeding because every chemical she was trying to remove would pass through to her infant.

Before pregnancy, a woman should clean up any potential toxins in her environment, including cleaning products, beauty products, and chemicals at work.

Many toxins in our environment act like hormones in our bodies, and cause imbalances in our natural hormones.[4] Environmental toxins contribute to rising rates of menstrual problems and infertility.[5] Identifying hormone imbalance before pregnancy not only helps fertility, it helps maintain the pregnancy and sets up the infant's own hormone system.

Although estrogen and progesterone are critical for pregnancy, there are other hormones such as thyroid hormones and adrenal hormones that, if imbalanced, can have profound negative effects on a baby. When I conduct my preconception workshops, I recommend women have laboratory evaluations for several key health issues, including proper hormone balance. One woman found that she had low thyroid hormone (hypothyroidism). A normal thyroid hormone level is critical for the physical growth and normal intellectual development of the child beginning in utero.[6] Just by identifying and treating this one hormone deficiency, she has improved her health and the future health of her child. All it took was a blood test.

Inflammation

Another key area to address before pregnancy is chronic inflammation. It is a common pathway for many diseases like autism, heart disease, and cancer. Inflammation is ongoing injury to body tissues at the cellular level. Poor diet and lack of nutrition leads to free radicals and oxidative stress in cells that causes inflammation. For digestion, probiotics regulate the immune system to decrease inflammation. Toxins cause inflammation through the creation of free radicals. Making positive changes in all three areas of the Triangle of Prevention ultimately reduces inflammation.

Timing

I recommend that all women take the time needed to evaluate and improve their health before pregnancy. An ideal time to start is 6 to 12 months before trying to get pregnant. Three months might be adequate for a woman without any health issues and who does not need to detoxify.

Women should review their particular risk factors with their medical professional and take actions to increase their chances of having a healthy child. This preconception stage is a perfect time for making steady changes and for detoxifying.

Summary

Unfortunately we live in a world that continually exposes us to a multitude of chemicals with unknown health consequences. We do know that a developing child, because of their small size and developing organs, is especially vulnerable. A woman before pregnancy has the opportunity to minimize her exposure and her infant's future exposure. This is the only time to detoxify and is very important for the prevention of autism.

42

Preconception health is not currently a focus of our nation's health system. Given the significant impact that the mother's health has on the health of her future baby (and the great costs of having a child with major health issues), investing in a mother's health before pregnancy is not only good common sense but also good financial sense. We should call on our nation's health policy makers to make preconception health a priority. We should call on our health insurers to make the smart business decision that prevention pays.

REFERENCES CHAPTER 4

1. Schorah CJ, Smithells RW. Primary prevention of neural tube defects with folic acid. *BMJ.* 1993;306(6885):1123-1124. DH19.

2. Thompson MD, Cole DE, Ray JG. Vitamin B-12 and neural tube defects: the Canadian experience. *Am J Clin Nutr.* 2009;89(2):697S-701S. DH20.

3. Arnold GL, Hyman SL, Mooney RA, Kirby RS. Plasma amino acids profiles in children with autism: potential risk of nutritional deficiencies. *J Autism Dev Disord.* 2003 Aug;33(4):449-54. DH393.

4. De Coster S, van Larebeke N. Endocrine-Disrupting Chemicals: Associated Disorders and Mechanisms of Action. *J of Env and Public Health.* Volume 2012 (2012), Article ID 713696, 52 pgs. DH394.

5. Ibid.

6. Henrichs J, Bongers-Schokking JJ, Schenk JJ, Ghassabian A, Schmidt HG, Visser TJ, Hooijkaas H, de Muinck Keizer-Schrama SM, Hofman A, Jaddoe VV, Visser W, Steegers EA, Verhulst FC, de Rijke YB, Tiemeier H. Maternal thyroid function during early pregnancy and cognitive functioning in early childhood: the generation R study. *J Clin Endocrinol Metab.* 2010 Sep;95(9):4227-34. DH410.

5

Optimizing Nutrition

A mother's nutritional status at the time of conception and during the first few weeks of pregnancy is crucial for ensuring a baby's healthy growth and development. From the very start, the developing fetus requires the basic building blocks needed to properly grow and develop.

The best time for a prospective mother to develop healthy eating habits is before pregnancy. It takes effort to change from a diet full of processed foods to an ideal diet of whole, organic foods. Most people make changes in eating patterns slowly and in small steps. Time is also needed for women to build up nutritional stores to be able to support a healthy pregnancy. Any effort toward a healthier diet is a positive change.

Healthy Nutrition Overview

Nutrition includes foods from our diet and vitamin/mineral supplements. This chapter will focus on the diet part of good nutrition including what to eat and what not to eat. The next chapter discusses targeted supplements for women before pregnancy.

The body breaks all food into protein, carbohydrates, and fats. Everyone needs a combination of all three. Complete proteins are important whether from meat and dairy or a combination of non-animal proteins. Complex carbohydrates include whole grains, plus a mix of vegetables and fruits totaling about 9 servings per day. Yes, the days of recommending 5 per day are long gone. We need as many antioxidants as possible from fruits and vegetables to combat all the stress we encounter from our environment. My family has greatly increased our fruit and vegetable intake by using a high-powered blender to make good-tasting smoothies.

The right fats are required for good health. To most people, essential fatty acids mean cod liver oil or fish oil. Yet these oils only contain omega-3 fats. Our bodies need two types of essential fatty acids: omega-3 (alpha-linolenic acid) and omega-6 (linoleic acid). Both are important for brain development and function. The omega-3 fatty acids are further broken-down in the body into two fats: docosahexaenoic acid (DHA) and eicosapentaenoic acid (EPA), both of which are found in fish and cod liver oils. DHA is important for visual and neurological development, while EPA decreases inflammation in the body. Our bodies also need omega-6 fats but we have an overabundance of omega-6 fatty acids in our American diet compared to omega-3 fatty acids. Therefore, as we will discuss in the next chapter, most women need to supplement omega-3 fatty acids since they are so crucial for an infant's brain development.

Organic Foods

Organic foods are grown without pesticides, genetically modified ingredients, growth hormones, or antibiotics. An animal product is considered organic if neither the animal nor its food has been treated with any of these substances.

When comparing organic food to mass-produced conventional foods, it is easy to see the difference. Organic foods often are richer in color and contain more nutrients.[1] However, since they have no preservatives, they sometimes have a shorter shelf life.

Although organic foods are more expensive, for the protection of a child's nervous system development, I would include organic foods as a critical part of the plan to prevent autism and ADHD. The Environmental Working Group website (www.ewg.org) has lists of the fruits and vegetables with the most pesticides and those with the least. If a woman cannot afford an all-organic diet, she should avoid the foods with the highest amount of pesticides.

Concerns with Non-organic Foods

Pesticides

The chemicals used on crops to kill insects and other pests come from families of compounds called *organochlorines* and *organophosphates*. These chemicals deposit in our fatty tissues, making it difficult for our bodies to eliminate them. They also disrupt hormones in our bodies and are toxic to the nervous system, especially a young child's developing nervous system. Several studies have compared pesticide exposure rates in pregnant women. Women with higher pesticide exposure had children with an increased incidence of autism and ADHD.[2,3,4]

Lack of nutrients

Foods get many of their nutrients from the soil in which they grow. If the soil is used repeatedly, the nutrient content becomes depleted. Organic farms, however, rotate and combine crops along with using mulch to improve the nutrients levels in the food.

Antibiotics

Antibiotics are often used in the meat and dairy industry, giving us continuing exposure to these drugs. When we are exposed to these antibiotics, the good bacteria (probiotics) in our intestines are destroyed. This allows other bacteria and infectious agents, such as viruses and yeast, to grow more easily and cause health problems.

Growth hormones

Growth hormones are often given to agricultural animals to increase their size and their milk supply. When consuming non-organic meat and dairy foods, we are exposed to this hormone along with pes-

47

ticides that disrupt our own hormones. We are now seeing long-term effects from these hormone disruptors including: infertility, increasing cancer rates, more birth defects involving the genitalia of infants, and earlier puberty in children. Obviously, these are major concerns.

Whole Foods

Whole foods are foods that exist in their natural state. Because the word whole means entire, whole foods contain all the necessary nutrition provided by nature. An optimal diet should contain as much whole foods as possible.

Not sure if the food is a whole food? Just read the ingredients. If a person can't understand, recognize, or pronounce an ingredient, it is not a whole food. Many preservatives, flavor enhancers, and dyes added to foods are chemicals. We do not recognize their names as foods because they are not foods. Yet these chemicals are put in many processed foods and are eaten every day.

Foods that start as whole foods can be processed so their form is not as nutritious. Nothing is added but nutrients have been removed by processing. Fruit juice is a good example of an altered whole food. A fruit, such as an apple, is a whole food. However, when you squeeze the juice from the apple, it is no longer a whole food. The juice may have some of the vitamins, but it loses some of the fiber and other nutritious parts of the apple such as *pectin*, a substance that helps bind the fruit cells together. This can make a difference in how much nutrition the body receives from the food and how it affects metabolism. The fruit sugar in a raw apple doesn't cause blood sugar to rise too quickly; the fiber and pectin in the apple slow the blood sugar down. However, apple juice does not have fiber and pectin causing the blood sugar to spike. Most processed fruit juices contain too much sugar and lack the full nutrition that would be gained from eating the whole fruit.

Clean Water

Water from the tap can contain many potential chemical contaminants including chlorine, fluoride, pesticides, and residues from pharmaceutical drugs. Most bottled water comes from municipal water supplies and is not well regulated. Women planning to get pregnant need to find out what is in their drinking water. They can ask for a report from their local water supplier or test their water with a home kit.

Filters

After learning what is in the water, the next step is figure out what type of filtering system is needed. Some refrigerators have pre-installed carbon filter systems in their water dispensers. Carbon filter pitchers are also available. Complete filters with reverse osmosis systems can also be installed under the sink or for the entire house. Because water is so integral to life and we need to drink several glasses a day, the small amount of toxins in our everyday water adds up over time and should be removed.

Chlorine

It is also important to address the issue of chlorine in bathing water. Chlorine has byproducts that can be carcinogenic. These byproducts are inhaled and absorbed by the skin during bathing. To eliminate this problem, shower and bath chlorine filters or whole house systems are available.

Diet Essentials

The following are important for proper nutrition and toxin avoidance:

- Complete proteins
- Complex carbohydrates (many vegetables and some fruits: at least 9 servings per day)
- Essential fatty acids
- Whole foods
- Organic foods
- Clean water

Foods to Avoid

Just as important as what to eat, is what not to eat. There are so many chemicals in processed food that it would be a stretch to even call them food. For example, most food colorings are made from petroleum. Many Americans predominately eat these processed, non-natural foods. These processed foods not only lack the nutrition of real foods, they contain ingredients foreign to the body.

The big offenders can be placed into several groups including: genetically modified foods (called GMs or GMOs), sugar, high fructose corn syrup, artificial sweeteners, trans fats, food dyes, food additives, and monosodium glutamate (MSG).

Genetically Modified Foods

A food is genetically modified (GM) when new DNA is put into a cell of a plant. After the plant has grown, all the cells of the plant will have the new DNA. The four main GM crops are soy, corn, cotton, and canola.

GM foods are made to benefit the businesses involved in food production. There are no known health benefits. There have been no long-term safety studies concerning the effects of GM foods on humans. However, researcher Jeffrey M. Smith has written several excellent resources on GM foods, including *Seeds of Deception*, where he describes serious concerns:

- *The new DNA codes for a new protein, which may be different in the plant than what is expected and therefore may act differently in the environment.*

- *The new protein may be harmful to people and may cause allergies.*

- *Since GM crops are made to be more tolerant of herbicides, it stands to reason that more herbicides will be sprayed and then remain on these crops. People will then be exposed to more herbicides on their foods.*

- *The final and most frightening concern is that the genes transferred into the crops will be then transferred into our genes. Food first goes into our intestines, where we have many bacteria. The new genes then can be transferred into those bacteria.*

Because of the lack of research and the above concerns, several European countries have banned GM foods. As a precaution, I recommend that women considering pregnancy avoid GM foods. Only a product labeled "No GM (or GMO) foods" can be considered safe.

Sugar

There are two primary sweeteners used in foods in the U.S.: (1) table sugar or sucrose and (2) high fructose corn syrup. Both sweeteners add calories without nutritional value. Most people can identify sources of sugar in desserts such as cookies and candy. But sugar also hides in many beverages, including juices, and in breakfast cereals (even those labeled organic, whole-grains, or gluten-free). Sugar is also in many condiments, such as ketchup, and many processed foods including breads and frozen foods.

The Downside of Sugar: Lick the Sugar Habit by Nancy Appleton, PhD, lists 76 negative effects of sugar. Below are the problems with sugar that would be most concerning to someone preparing for a healthy pregnancy and a healthy child.

Depletes nutrition

In a study of children ranging in age from 13 months to 9 years, those with low sugar intake had a higher intake of protein, fiber, and good fats than children with a high sugar intake.[5] The low sugar group also had a higher intake of beneficial vitamin E, niacin (vitamin B3), calcium, and zinc.

The dietary goal before pregnancy is to maximize nutrition stores in order to have a healthy baby. Substituting sugar for healthy foods just does not make sense. Many children with autism have severe nutritional deficiencies.

Other studies have shown that sugar depletes minerals including chromium,[6] which is needed for blood sugar regulation, and affects the body's levels of calcium, magnesium, and copper. Having good mineral status before, during, and after pregnancy is one of the best ways to give a child a good start on health.

Suppresses the immune system

Sugar damages the function of white blood cells and decreases some nutrients, such as zinc, which are needed for proper immune function. Therefore, sugar consumption increases the risk of infection. People correlate winter with the cold and flu season; however these illnesses also correlate with the holiday season, which often begins with Halloween and a large increase in the consumption of sugar.

Increases yeast and harmful bacteria in the intestine

A large percentage of children with autism have an imbalance of good and bad bacteria – called *dysbiosis*.[7] Yeast often plays a role in this condition. Yeast thrives on sugar. So to keep the digestive system (and its important immunity function) in balance, sugar intake should be greatly reduced.

Triggers negative effects on mood and behavior

Sugar in the body causes large swings in blood sugar. These spikes in blood sugar cause the body to release the hormone insulin. Insulin then causes the blood sugar to drop and can result in hypoglycemia. The drop in blood sugar causes a craving for sugar and the cycle continues. Rapid changes in blood sugar cause shifts in mood from inattention to irritability.

Increases inflammation in the body

When a high intake of sugar leads to a high level of insulin in the body, this can cause inflammation. Inflammation injures the tissues and is a key factor in many chronic diseases, including autism, diabetes, and heart disease among others.

Cutting Back on Sugar

Reducing sugar intake is one of the more difficult dietary changes to make, but for a woman's health and her future baby it is essential. The goal is to decrease sugar intake to less than 10 teaspoons (50 grams) a day, but no more than 15 teaspoons (75 grams). Food labels list the number of grams of sugar per serving. Five grams of sugar is roughly equivalent to 1 teaspoon of sugar. Considering that one glass of orange juice often contains about 30 grams or 6 teaspoons of sugar, the teaspoons add up quickly. By eating cold cereal with milk and orange juice for breakfast, it is easy obtain the recommended daily sugar intake in just one meal.

High Fructose Corn Syrup

High fructose corn syrup is a processed sugar and therefore not a natural or whole food. Manufacturers use high fructose corn syrup because it is less expensive than regular table sugar. Fructose is a natural sugar found in fruit in low concentrations. It is also made naturally when sucrose or table sugar is broken-down in the body into glucose and fructose. These natural sugars are very different than the artificially created high fructose corn syrup. The amount of fructose in high fructose corn syrup is much higher than would be found in whole foods, and the body doesn't naturally know what to do with this excess fructose.

High fructose corn syrup is primarily consumed through sodas and other sweetened beverages that were once sweetened with sugar. High fructose corn syrup is also hidden in many other processed foods such as breads, packaged meals, crackers, peanut butter, jellies, and even condiments such as ketchup. Because there is no nutritional value to high fructose corn syrup, people miss out on all the good nutrition they would have consumed when eating other nutritious foods.

Negative health effects of high fructose corn syrup

Like sucrose or table sugar, high fructose corn syrup causes the body to lose minerals as it tries to process the sweetener. These minerals, such as calcium, magnesium, and zinc, are important for health and are often low in diets, especially in children with autism.

High fructose corn syrup also creates unique health concerns. Fructose is metabolized by the liver. Research studies have shown an association with high fructose corn syrup and an increase in nonalcoholic fatty liver disease.[8] The excess fat stored in the liver impairs its function. Because the liver is one of the primary organs that help the body detoxify chemicals, anything that negatively affects the liver could impair the body's ability to detoxify harmful substances.

High fructose corn syrup may also interfere with copper metabolism by hindering a copper-dependent enzyme called *lysyl oxidase*.[9] This enzyme is needed to form collagen and elastin, which are integral to many of the structural tissues in the body such as the skin. Fructose appears to damage the development of collagen and elastin in growing animals.

Artificial Sweeteners: Aspartame and Sucralose

The two main artificial sweeteners used in the U.S. today are aspartame and sucralose. They are both manufactured chemicals that do not exist in nature and therefore are not whole foods.

Aspartame

Aspartame is the artificial sweetener found in Nutrasweet™ and Equal™. The chemical name is 1-aspartyl 1-phenylalanine methyl ester. It is made primarily of two amino acids, phenylalanine and aspartic acid. While these two amino acids exist in our food supply, they do not naturally occur together or in high amounts.

Studies have shown that the chemicals in aspartame have the potential to cause negative health effects by reducing the antioxidant glutathione.[10] When consumed in high quantities, they act as *excitotoxins* and can damage the nervous system. This is especially true of aspartic acid. Excitotoxins increase the firing of cells in the nervous system, thereby causing the system to become overactive. This response is particularly dangerous to the developing nervous system in unborn babies and young children.

Also of concern is the fact that aspartame contains a methyl ester, which is absorbed into the body as methanol—a wood alcohol or paint remover. The methanol itself is then converted in the body to formaldehyde. Both methanol and formaldehyde are toxic substances, not foods found in nature and meant to be eaten.

Given the above adverse health effects and the competition with sucralose (described below), aspartame is being used less and less in foods.

Sucralose

Sucralose is the primary artificial sweetener used in food products in the U.S. today and is found in Splenda™. It is a chlorinated artificial sugar with a chemical name 1,6-dichloro-1,6-dideoxy-beta-D-fructofuranosyl-4-chloro-4-deoxy-alpha-D-galactopyranoside. There is no food found in nature with a name like that!

Sucralose was accidentally discovered to be sweet in an industrial chemical lab. Sucralose is made by combining chlorine with a carbon-containing sugar, thereby making it an organochlorine. Organochlorines are also used as an active toxic ingredient in insecticides.

Because sucralose is a newer artificial sweetener, less is known about its effects on people. No studies have been done on pregnant women or children; however, other organochlorines and organophosphate pesticides cause damage to unborn children and young children. In addition, organochlorine exposure during pregnancy has been shown to increase the risk of autism.[11] Metabolic studies in animals using sucralose have shown a concentrating affect in the mouse fetus and also problems with sucralose excretion.[12] Sucralose can also trigger headaches, especially in people prone to migraines.[13]

A 2008 article[14] in the *Journal of Toxicology and Environmental Health* identified two further concerns of sucralose: (1) the sweetener decreases the amount of good bacteria in the intestine and (2) it alters the body's ability to detoxify chemicals.

The other concern is that sucralose alters two enzymes that are important for our body to detoxify: intestinal p-glycoprotein and cytochrome p-450. Altering the body's ability to detoxify can interfere with how other drugs and toxins are absorbed and processed in the body.

Trans Fats

Trans fats are made by adding hydrogen to a food to make the fat more stable and ensure a longer shelf life. Any food that has hydrogenated or partially hydrogenated oils contains trans fats. These fats can also be made by deep frying foods and damaging the oils. Trans fats are not whole foods. Luckily, trans fat levels are now required to be part of food labels for easy identification. Given the negative health effects of fried foods and hydrogenated oils, efforts are also under way to ban foods containing trans fats.

Trans fats have negative health effects. The omega-3 fatty acid DHA is very important to neurological health and is essential during fetal development and early childhood. However, trans fats replace DHA in the brain cells. They can also block the body's ability to convert essential fats into omega-3 fatty acids that are needed by the brain.

Neurologic health is compromised in unborn children and infants when the trans fats from the mother are passed through the placenta and breast milk.[15] The amount of trans fats a child receives depends upon the mother's diet. In addition, a mother that has a higher intake of trans fats tends to have a lower intake of the essential fatty acids.[16] This can have a significant negative impact on the child including lower birth weight and a poorer neurological exam at 18 months of age.[17] Studies of fatty acid and trans fat levels in umbilical cord blood have shown that infants with the lowest levels of trans fats and the highest levels of DHA have the best neurological exams as toddlers.[18]

To compound problems, trans fats are also pro-inflammatory, which means they increase oxidative stress and inflammation markers in the body. These processes are associated with most chronic diseases and aging. This includes autism in which there are high levels of oxidative stress.[19]

Food Additives

Approximately 3,000 food additives have been approved by the Food and Drug Administration (FDA) and more are approved each year. There have been no long-term studies on the safety of these food additives on developing infants and children. Nor have there been studies on the safety of combining these additives, which is what happens in real life when we eat a variety of foods. Two specific types of food additives of concern are food dyes made from petroleum and food preservatives that prevent contamination from bacteria.

There are several preservatives to specifically watch out for and avoid. These include sulfites and any form of benzoate: benzoic acid, calcium benzoate, and potassium benzoate. Sulfites can cause many allergic symptoms, especially in people with asthma.[20] Butylated hydroxyanisole (BHA), the related compound butylated hydroxtoluene (BHT), and nitrites affect the cellular level and have been shown to increase the risk of cancer.[21]

Negative health effects of food additives

Food additives create the following health concerns:

Increased hyperactivity

Several decades ago, Dr. Benjamin Feingold discovered that food dyes, food additives, and salicylates increase hyperactivity. He instituted the Feingold diet, which is free of these preservatives. Eliminating these foods also decreases symptoms such as headaches, stomach pains, and temper tantrums. Subsequent studies have shown that these preservatives, in addition to sodium benzoate, increase hyperactive behavior in children with or without ADHD.[22]

Allergic symptoms

Allergies are commonly seen after ingestion of food additives, especially in children and adults prone to allergies. Two specific food additives, the food dye tartrazine and sulfite preservatives, commonly trigger wheezing in people with asthma. The intake of food dyes, food preservatives, and citric acid causes a host of other allergic symptoms in children such as increased rates of asthma, eczema, runny nose (rhinitis), hives, and gastrointestinal symptoms. Food dyes have even triggered cases of multiple chemical sensitivity and anaphylactic shock in children.[23]

Negative nutrients

Food dyes and additives are actually negative nutrients much like sugar and high fructose corn syrup. Instead of adding good nutrients, such as vitamins or minerals, they can cause a loss of minerals. Tartrazine and other food dyes have been found to increase the amount of zinc excreted in the urine.[24] Zinc is a critical element for the nervous system.

MSG and Other Glutamates

Monosodium glutamate (MSG) and other forms of glutamate are chemicals used in foods to enhance the taste and sell more food. Again, these substances are not added for our health benefit. Glutamates can be found in many processed foods including soups and snack foods such as chips, packaged meals, canned food, salad dressings, and candy.

Government regulation states that foods have to be labeled as having MSG only if they contain 100% MSG. Therefore many packaged foods will have other names for food additives that contain some MSG or other glutamates, such as:

- Hydrolyzed vegetable protein
- Other hydrolyzed proteins such as plant, soy, textured, or protein isolate

- Sodium or calcium caseinate
- Yeast extracts and many types of flavoring, including "natural" flavoring

Any packaged food that has an ingredient that cannot be identified as a whole food may contain some MSG or other glutamates.

Negative health effects

MSG and glutamates cause detrimental effects on the nervous system.

Excitotoxins

Glutamate is a natural neurotransmitter in the brain that causes excitation or activation of the brain cells. When additional glutamate is added to the body from food, the brain becomes over excited. The brain cells start firing and cannot turn off. With continuing exposure, eventually cells cannot fire anymore and die.

All humans are vulnerable to the effects of excitotoxic glutamates. But some groups of people are much more susceptible than others, and children are one of the most susceptible. The brain has its largest growth from the third trimester of pregnancy through the second year of life. During this time, the immature growing brain is 4 times more sensitive to excitotoxic glutamates than a more fully developed brain. Excitotoxic glutamates cross the placenta during pregnancy and pass into breast milk during nursing. Because newborn babies may not have a fully developed blood brain barrier, they receive a higher concentration of excitotoxic glutamates than an older child or an adult.[25, 26]

Inflammation

Microglia, which are specialized cells in the brain, are an important part of the brain's immune system. These cells are sensitive to glutamates. When microglia are activated, they release chemicals called *cytokines*, which cause inflammation in the brain. Once the microglia cells are activated, they continue to release cytokines. This activity causes chronic inflammation in the brain, as seen in children with autism.

Antioxidant depletion

Antioxidant enzymes help prevent cell damage and death. Like the other systems, newborns do not have a fully developed antioxidant enzyme system. Excitotoxic glutamates further deplete some of these antioxidant enzymes, making it harder for young bodies to prevent inflammation. In the first few years of life, when the brain is still developing, young children are at a significant risk of neurologic damage from excitotoxins.

Disease associated with excess glutamates

Many diseases are associated with excess glutamates. Autism is the primary related chronic disorder in children. Alzheimer's, Parkinson's disease, Huntington's chorea, and amyotrophic lateral sclerosis (ALS or Lou Gerhig's disease) are all related chronic disorders in adults. Inflammation of the brain cells is common in autism and Alzheimer's. Acute disorders associated with excess excitotoxic glutamates include seizures, migraines, depression, and anxiety.[27]

Protection from MSG and glutamates

Women should avoid MSG and other glutamates in food as much as possible. They should have a good intake of the following nutrients that are neuroprotective and guard against excitotoxic damage:

- Zinc
- Magnesium
- Taurine—an amino acid needed for better magnesium absorption
- Docosahexaenoic acid (DHA)—a fatty acid

These nutrients are often low in adults, including women considering pregnancy, and in children with autism, making the children more susceptible to glutamate damage.

Foods to Avoid

- Genetically modified foods (GMs)
- High fructose corn syrup
- Artificial sweeteners (sucralose with trademark Splenda, Aspartame)

- Trans fats
- Food dyes
- Food preservatives (benzoic acid, calciumbenzonate, potassium benzoate, BHA, BHT, nitrites and sulfites)
- MSG or foods with monosodium glutamate

Summary

We make many, many decisions every day about what to eat and what not to eat. Depending on the foods we choose, we can give our bodies vitamins, minerals, proteins, and good fats. Or we can give our bodies substances that in many cases were actually created in a laboratory and rob us of nutrition. The chemicals in artificial foods act upon us in many negative ways.

Diet changes are challenging, but they are worth the effort. For optimum health and for healthy babies, whole foods and organic foods are vital.

CHAPTER 5 REFERENCES

1. Crinnion W. Organic foods contain higher levels of certain nutrients, lower levels of pesticides and may provide health benefits for the consumer. *Alt Med Review.* 2010;15(1):4-12. DH332.

2. Eskenazi B, Huen K, Marks A, Harley KG, Bradman A, Barr DB, Holland N. PON1 and neurodevelopment in children from the CHAMACOS study exposed to organophosphate pesticides in utero. *Environ Health Perspect.* 2010 Dec;118(12):1775-81. DH231.

3. Rauh V, Arunajadai S, Horton M, Perera F, Hoepner L, Barr DB, Whyatt R. Seven-year neurodevelopmental scores and prenatal exposure to chlorpyrifos, a common agricultural pesticide. *Environ Health Perspect.* 2011 Aug;119(8):1196-201. DH431.

4. Marks AR, Harley K, Bradman A, Kogut K, Barr DB, Johnson C, Calderon N, Eskenazi B. Organophosphate pesticide exposure and attention in young Mexican-American children: the CHAMACOS study. *Environ Health Perspect.* 2010 Dec;118(12):1768-74. DH232.

5. Routtinen S, Niinikoski H, Lagstrom H, Ronnemaa T, Hakanen M, Viikari J, Jokinen E, Simell O. High sucrose intake is associated with poor quality of diet and growth between 13 months and 9 years of age: the special Turku Coronary

Risk Factor Intervention Project. *Pediatrics.* 2008 Jun;121(6):e1676-85. DH173.

6. Kozlovsky AS, Moser PB, Reiser S, Anderson RA. Effects of diets high in simple sugars on urinary chromium losses. *Metabolism.* 35 June 1986:515-18. DH218.

7. Horvath K, Perman JA. Autism and gastrointestinal symptoms. *Curr Gastroenterol Rep.* 2002;4(3):251-258. DH68.

8. Ouyang X et al. Fructose consumption as a risk factor for non-alcoholic fatty liver disease. *J Hepatol.* 2008 Jun;48(6):993-9. DH170.

9. Fields M, Ferretti RJ, Reiser S, Smith JC Jr. The severity of copper deficiency in rats is determined by the type of dietary carbohydrate. *Proceedings of the Society of Experimental Biology and Medicine.* 1984;175:530-537. DH156.

10. Abhilash M, Paul MV, Varghese MV, Nair RH. Effect of long term intake of aspartame on antioxidant defense status in liver. *Food Chem Toxicol.* 2011 Jun;49(6):1203-7. DH333.

11. Roberts EM, English PB, Grether JK, Windham GC, Somberg L, Wolff C. Maternal residence near agricultural pesticide applications and autism spectrum disorders among children in the California central valley. *Environmental Health Perspectives.* October 2007; 115(20):1482-1489. DM172.

12. Abou-Domia MB, El-Masry EM, Abdel-Rahman AA, McLendon RE, Schiffman SS. Splenda alters gut microflora and increases intestinal p-glycoprotein and cytochrome p-450 in male rats. *J Toxicol Environ Health.* 2008;71(21):1415-29. DH151.

13. Grotz VL. Sucralose and migraine. *Headache.* 2008 Jan;48(1):164-5. DH159.

14. Abou-Domia 2008.

15. Innis SM. Trans fatty intakes during pregnancy, infancy, and early childhood. *Atheroscler Suppl.* 2006;7(2):17-20. DH37.

16. Ibid.

17. Bouwstra H, Dijck-Brouwer J, Decsi T, Boehm G, Boersma ER, Muskiet FA, Hadders-Algra M. Neurologic condition of healthy term infants at 18 months: positive association with venous umbilical DHA status and negative association with umbilical trans-fatty acids. *Pediatr Res.* 2006;60(3):334-339. DH31.

18. Ibid.

19. James SJ, Cutler P, Melnyk S, Jernigan S, Janak L, Gaylor DW, Neubrander JA. Metabolic biomarkers of increased oxidative stress and impaired methyla-

tion capacity in children of autism. *Am J Clin Nutr.* 2004;80(6):1611-1617. DH118.

20. Stevenson DD, Simon RA. Sensitivity to ingested metabisulphites in asthmatic subjects. *J Allergy Clin Immunol.* 1981;68:26-32. DH175.

21. Taylor G. Nitrates, nitrites, nitrosamines and cancer. *Nutrition and Health.* 1983 2:1. DH225.

22. McCann D, Barrett A, Cooper A, Crumpler D, Dalen L, Grimshaw K, Kitchin E, Lok K, Porteous L, Prince E, Sonuga-Barke E, Warner JO, Stevenson. Food additives and hyperactive behavior in 3-year-old and 8/9-year-old children in the community: a randomized, double-blinded, placebo-controlled trial. *Lancet.* 2007 Nov 3;370(9598):1560-7. DH220.

23. Inomata N, Osuna H, Fujita H, Ogawa T, Ikezawa Z. Multiple chemical sensitivities following intolerance to azo dye in sweets in a 5-year-old girl. *Allergol Int.* 2006 Jun;55(2):203-5. DH161.

24. Ward NI, Soulsbury K, Zettel V, Colquhoun I, Bunday S, Barnes B. The influence of the chemical additive tartrazine on the zinc status of hyperactive children-a double blind placebo controlled study. *J of Nut Med.* 1 (1990);51057. DH180.

25. Blaylock R. Interaction of cytokines, excitotoxins, and reactive nitrogen and oxygen species in Autism spectrum disorders. *J Amer Nutr Assoc.* 2003, 6:21-35. DH153.

26. Blaylock R. *Excitotoxins: The Taste that Kills.* Health Press NA, Albuquerque, NM. 1997.

27. Ibid.

6

Nutrition Testing and Supplement Plan

In the last chapter we learned that many potential mothers have nutritional deficiencies which can lead to health problems later on for the child (including autism and ADHD). The best time to address proper nutrition is before pregnancy. In this chapter we will cover the best ways of testing for specific nutritional deficiencies and how to overcome these deficiencies—including the use of supplements.

Obviously it would be ideal if we could get all the nutrients we need from our food. The problem is that much of our food is grown in depleted soil and highly processed, so it is not as nourishing as it used to be. Since most Americans also do not eat a balanced diet, supplements are needed for the majority of people but especially for women planning to have a baby.

Prenatal Vitamins

Research shows that women who take prenatal vitamins throughout pregnancy have healthier babies.[1] These vitamins provide the mother with increased levels of specific vitamins such as iron. A recent study also shows that women who take a prenatal vitamin for the entire pregnancy may have a lower risk of having a child with autism.[2] Since the very beginning of the pregnancy is so important for the health of the child, I recommend that women begin taking a prenatal vitamin before she becomes pregnant.

We have known for a long time that woman who take folic acid has a lower chance of having a child with a neural tube defect, like spina bifida. The folic acid only helps if it is given in the very beginning of pregnancy. Many women do not know they are pregnant until 6 to 8 weeks, when the neural tube is already formed. Beginning folic acid at that point is too late.

If a woman is malnourished and begins a prenatal vitamin at the time of conception, it is still too late to overcome many nutritional deficiencies. For example, if a woman is low in vitamin D the amount in a prenatal vitamin will not be enough to correct this low level. The fetus could still be affected by the woman's deficiency even if she is taking a recommended amount of vitamin D from her prenatal vitamin. Therefore, it makes sense to evaluate a woman's diet and nutrition stores before she gets pregnant and supplement what is needed. High doses of supplements during pregnancy could potentially be harmful to a small developing fetus, so building nutrition stores with higher doses of vitamins and minerals is safer before pregnancy.

Even though prenatal vitamins provide an extra amount of the nutrient iron, they still fall short in several critical nutrients needed for a healthy pregnancy and healthy development of the infant. These include zinc, vitamin D, omega-3 fatty acids and for some women, calcium and magnesium. I also recommend special, more absorbable forms of some vitamins such as folinic acid or methylfolate for folic acid, and methyl B12 for vitamin B12. A few brands of prenatal vitamins contain these more absorbable forms.

Many of the specific nutrients described in Table 6-1 below have important roles in both a positive pregnancy outcome and a proper development of the baby's nervous system. We are also learning more about individual biochemistry and the fact that not all people require the same amount of a given vitamin or nutrient. Because of this fact, it is important to test for levels of some of these vitamins and minerals. This helps to determine nutrition supplement needs.

Table 6-1 - Special Dietary Supplements Recommended Before Pregnancy

Supplement	Recommended daily amount	Food and supplement sources
Prenatal vitamin	1 a day is essential!	Over the counter
Iron	Provided in prenatal vitamins. Total 45 to 60 mg (Depending on ferritin level)	Beef (and other red meats), chicken, kidney beans, cooked spinach, leafy greens, and blackstrap molasses
Zinc (in addition to prenatal vitamin)	15 mg Total: 30mg	Beef, lamb, oysters, seeds (sesame, pumpkin, sunflower), and beans (lima and kidney)
Vitamin D (in addition to prenatal vitamin)	1,000 to 3,000 IU (Depending on vitamin D level)	Cod liver oil, fish (salmon, mackerel, tuna, sardines), milk, egg, and Swiss cheese
Essential fatty acids, especially docosahexaenoic acid (DHA) (some prenatal vitamins have DHA but usually not enough)	Cod liver oil: 1 t DHA: 1,000 mg Mixed seeds: 1 T	Cod liver and flaxseed oil, seeds (flax, pumpkin, sunflower, sesame), and oily fish (sardines, anchovies, mackerel, salmon, herring)
Methylation vitamins (all prenatal vitamins have B vitamins but not all have these absorbable forms)	Folinic acid or methylfolate: 1,000 mcg (1 mg) Methyl B12: 1000 mcg (1 mg) (depending on homocysteine level)	Folinic acid: Fortified cereals, spinach, and great northern beans Methyl B12: Meat, eggs, and cheese

Abbreviations:
mg = milligram; IU = international units; t = teaspoon; T = tablespoon; mcg = micrograms

Iron

Red blood cells use iron to carry oxygen around the body. This is why people with low iron stores (called *anemia*) feel tired and short of breath. Adequate iron is important for having a healthy pregnancy and for the neurological health of the infant.

Iron benefits for pregnancy

During pregnancy, iron requirements increase because the mother is supporting oxygen needs for herself and her baby with an increased blood volume. Iron deficiency has been linked to many health conditions that affect both the mother and baby. Adequate iron levels before pregnancy will:

1. Reduce risk of infertility[3]
2. Ensure proper development of the placenta (which is critical in supporting a healthy pregnancy)
3. Ensure healthy birth weight
4. Reduce risk of preterm labor
5. Prevent postpartum depression

Benefits for children (relationship to autism)

Many children with autism and ADHD have low iron stores.[4,5] In one study the symptoms of ADHD were lessened after dietary levels of iron were increased.[6] Therefore, preventing low iron stores in babies and children is another way to prevent delayed neurologic development, subsequent symptoms of ADHD, and possibly symptoms of autism. Iron is also critical for the growth and normal neurologic development of babies and children.[7] A child with iron deficiency is also more likely to absorb and retain poisonous heavy metals such as lead.[8]

Sources

There are two forms of iron in food: heme and nonheme. *Heme iron*, which is found in meat (especially red meat), is the most easily absorbed. *Nonheme iron* is found in green leafy vegetables, and specific seeds, nuts and herbs. Iron is also found in black strap molasses, which I craved when I was pregnant. People may even ingest iron after by using a cast iron cooking pot. Iron is best absorbed with foods containing vitamin C.

Testing

Because iron is such an important nutrient for pregnancy and breastfeeding, a woman's iron levels should be measured before pregnancy. Many health practitioners will measure the complete blood count (CBC) and look at two tests: hemoglobin and hematocrit. But these tests do not show problems with iron until iron levels are much lower indicating a person has true anemia. The ideal blood check for iron is a blood ferritin test. A ferritin level between 40 and 70 µg/L meets the iron needs for a healthy pregnancy and an adequate supply in breast milk (table 6-2).

Supplements

Most women should take an iron-fortified prenatal vitamin to get extra iron. However, if her levels of ferritin are elevated, then a woman should check back with her doctor before taking this supplement.

It is important not to take iron at the same time as other minerals such as zinc because they compete for absorption. Since most women will get their iron from prenatal vitamins, they should take their other minerals such as zinc and calcium at other times of the day.

Zinc

Zinc is another mineral that is critical for pregnancy, nursing, and a baby's healthy development. Insufficient zinc, which is among the most common nutritional deficiencies in the U.S., is associated with both female and male infertility.

Benefits in pregnancy

Adequate zinc may reduce the risk of pregnancy and labor complications, reduce child morbidity, and support child growth.[9,10]

Benefits in children (relationship to autism)

In my practice, the vast majority of children with autism, including those with attention deficit and sensory issues, have low zinc reserves. Zinc is crucial for brain development, cognition, immune function, and the ability to taste foods. Children with autism often experience problems in these areas.

Children with autism cannot interpret the world around them correctly because their brains are not functioning at a healthy level. They have problems regulating their moods, so every day is a roller coaster. Zinc helps the brain function and process information to learn. There is a saying in biomedical autism training: "No zinc, no think." I frequently say this to parents because it summarizes the importance of zinc.

Children with autism have many documented deficits in their immune system that cause chronic infections and slow healing. The digestive system is often affected, leading to chronic diarrhea and an even greater loss of zinc. This creates a vicious cycle of zinc deficiency, a poor immune system, chronic infections, diarrhea, and further zinc deficiency. Ensuring adequate levels of zinc to strengthen the immune system and avoid chronic infections is another important aspect of preventing autism. Children who receive zinc supplements experience improvement in mood, attention, and learning. They also have better appetites and have a more varied diet.

Sources

Like iron, zinc is found primarily in animal foods such as red meat. Zinc is also found in small quantities in some greens (chard), seeds (pumpkin and sunflower), and beans (lima and kidney).

Testing

Since zinc is one of the most common nutritional deficiencies, testing is helpful but not always necessary. During a physical exam there are signs for identifying a zinc deficiency. A classic sign is horizontal white lines on the fingernails. Since zinc also affects the skin, stretch marks are also a sign (although other problems can also cause these marks). Whether signs are present or not, I recommend all women take extra zinc before pregnancy. All prospective fathers should also take zinc supplements before pregnancy since zinc is one of the most important nutrients for male fertility.

The best test for zinc is a blood test where the zinc level is measured in the red blood cell. The normal range is 70 to 120 ug/dL. An optimal level before pregnancy is 100 to 120 ug/dL. If a zinc test is ordered without specifying it is for the red blood cell, the lab will run the test to measure plasma zinc, which is less accurate. Because zinc is circulated in the blood but stored in the body, a plasma zinc test does not give a good estimate of the total zinc stores. This is also true for many other minerals. If I cannot get a red blood cell zinc level test because of lab limitations, I will look at a plasma zinc level and if it is in the bottom third of normal levels, then zinc stores are lower than they should be, and zinc supplementation is needed. If blood plasma zinc levels are below normal, I know that zinc stores are very low.

Supplements

The general recommended daily intake of zinc for women in child-bearing years is 15 mg/day. Optimal intake for most women who are pregnant is 30 mg/day (Table 6-1). Most prenatal vitamins provide only partial zinc requirements, so I recommend an additional 15 mg/day of zinc in a form that is easy to absorb such as zinc picolinate or a zinc chelate.

Too much zinc may induce a copper deficiency. This can lead to anemia in much the same way as an iron deficiency. However, this is usually not a problem and should not be a reason to avoid extra zinc supplements. Optimal zinc levels of 30 mg/day during pregnancy are generally not high enough to affect copper absorption. Since many people, including children with autism, have copper levels that are too high, extra zinc is normally not a problem.

Vitamin D

Vitamin D is a fat-soluble vitamin known for building and maintaining strong bones. Yet bone growth is only one function of vitamin D. There are vitamin D receptors on every cell in the body. Vitamin D acts more like a hormone than a typical vitamin or mineral and is unique in that the primary source is from the sun and not food. Its functions range from stimulating the release of insulin from the pancreas (thus controlling blood sugar), to regulating cell growth, to decreasing allergies and autoimmune tendencies (such as Type 1 diabetes).

Benefits in pregnancy

Optimal levels of vitamin D are essential during pregnancy. Low levels of vitamin D during pregnancy are associated with numerous problems including:

1. Low infant birth weight
2. Insulin resistance and gestational diabetes, both of which affect blood sugar in the mom and baby
3. Increased risk of asthma, immune and allergic disorders in children

Benefits in children (relationship to autism)

I have consistently found low levels of vitamin D in children, whether or not they have autism. This seems to be a trend in our country that is caused by excessive sun avoidance, the use of sun blocks to prevent skin cancer, and decreased intake of dietary vitamin D. Recent research on healthy infants and toddlers shows that 12% of young children had full vitamin D deficiency and 40% had levels that were suboptimal.[11]

Another recent study found that vitamin D deficiency might be a trigger for autism.[12]

Immune and allergic disorders are increasingly found in children, especially children with autism. Adequate levels of vitamin D help decrease autoimmune and allergic tendencies including the risk of type 1 diabetes.[13]

Sources

Sun exposure is the best source of vitamin D. However, people are now wary of sunburn and risk for subsequent skin cancer. In addition, sunscreen drastically decreases the body's ability to make the vitamin. Food sources of vitamin D in this country are limited mainly to fortified dairy products (table 6-1). Many dairy milk substitutes, such as soy, rice, and almond milk, are now fortified with calcium and vitamin D. Some cod liver oils have vitamin D, but most fish oils have inadequate levels.

Actually, the best way to get vitamin D is from brief exposure to sunlight. Just 10 minutes in the sun with a tank top will provide 10,000 IUs of vitamin D.

Testing

Vitamin D is easy to measure in a blood test. It is important to measure 25-hydroxy (25-OH) vitamin D, which changes into the most active form of the vitamin. Full vitamin deficiency occurs at a level of <20 ng/mL. Recommendations by the general medical community are for optimal levels >30 ng/mL. Vitamin D experts recommend levels between 50 to 80 ng/mL based on research of healthy people living in sun-rich environments. Vitamin D toxicity is seen at levels >150 ng/mL and sometimes not until the level reaches 200 ng/mL.

Supplements

For women considering pregnancy, I recommend having their 25-OH vitamin D levels checked. If the levels are <40 ng/mL, I would supplement with 4,000 IU/day of vitamin D; if the levels are >40 ng/mL, I recommend that supplement with a minimum of 2,000 IU/day. If levels are above 80, I recommend women check with their doctor.

Essential Fatty Acids

Our bodies cannot produce omega-3 and omega-6 fatty acids on their own, which is why they are called essential fatty acids. Therefore, we need to get both of these essential fats from our diet. In the U.S. most people consume sufficient quantities of omega-6 fatty acids, but not enough omega-3.

The body converts the fatty acids as follows:
<u>Step 1</u>: *Omega-3-* Alpha-linolenic acid (ALA) converted to eicosapentaenoic acid (EPA) and docosahexaenoic acid (DHA) in the body.
<u>Step 2</u>: *Omega-6-* Linoleic acid (LA) converted to gamma-linolenic acid (GLA) and then arachidonic acid (AA) in the body.

There are people who take flax seed oil to obtain their omega-3 fats. The problem is that not all people can convert the ALA in flax to DHA and EPA. With the high need for DHA in the infant's brain, the only safe way for women to obtain this is by taking a source of DHA directly.

Benefits of omega-3 fatty acids in pregnancy

It is well known that the essential omega-3 fats are good for health including the heart, brain, and joints. Importantly, omega-3 fat DHA is also essential to an infant's brain growth. The brain is 60% fat and the infant needs these fats to grow the brain properly beginning in pregnancy. The impact of a mother's intake of these essential fats cannot be underestimated in her infant's future health and the prevention of autism.

Importance of essential fats

- Needed for producing hormones that support pregnancy
- Reduces the chances of premature delivery
- Reduces post-partum depression

Benefits in children (relationship to autism)

Many studies have looked at a mother's intake of omega-3 fatty acids during pregnancy and its effect on infant development. Studies have shown higher IQs in infants who receive larger amounts of essential fats, especially DHA.[14] One research study compared the development of infants whose mothers took 4 gms/day fish oil (DHA and EPA combined) during the last half of pregnancy versus infants whose mothers took no fish oil.[15] Infants of mothers who took fish oil showed better development and learning skills in the following areas: speech, socialization, hearing, hand-eye coordination, and reasoning ability. These are all significant deficits in children with autism. Figure 4 in Chapter 3, The Power of Prevention, contains a list of many the positive studies about omega-3 fats and children's development. There is a preponderance of evidence for the importance of omega-3 fats in pregnant women and thus strong support for taking them beginning before pregnancy.

Sources of essential fatty acids

There are several animal and non-animal sources of essential fats. The primary animal source used to be the meat of grass-fed animals. Many animals are now grain-fed, and their meat has much higher amounts of saturated fats. Fish (especially cold water fish) have high levels of omega-3 fats. However, because farm-raised fish don't have a natural diet of algae, they have much lower levels of essential fats.

Eggs from chickens that have been fed special healthy diets can be a good source of essential fats. Fish oil and cod liver oil are good sources of the two essential fatty acids, particularly DHA and EPA. Women should consider the source before adding fish, fish oil, or cod liver oil to the diet. They should be careful to avoid the risks of contamination from mercury and polychlorinated biphenyls (PCBs), which are very harmful to the mother and baby.

Non-animal sources of essential fats include many types of seeds (table 6-1). Omega-3 fats are found in flax, pumpkin seeds, and walnuts. Omega-6 fats are found primarily in soybean, safflower, sunflower, corn, and sesame oils. All of those seeds and their oils contain some of both essential fatty acids. A tablespoon or more of a combination of these seeds is a good way to obtain additional essential fats.

Testing

The amount of essential fatty acids is usually measured by their level in red blood cells. Because levels of DHA and EPA in American women are universally low, it is not usually necessary to evaluate a woman's levels. What is necessary is an adequate intake of all essential fatty acids and extra DHA.

Supplements

In addition to a daily intake of seeds, I recommend one teaspoon/day of cod liver oil, which is a good source of DHA, EPA, and vitamins A and D (Table 6-1). However, too much vitamin A in the fat-soluble form found in cod liver oil may result in birth defects. The other of the omega-3 fats (including DHA and EPA) should be supplemented with fish oils.

Methylation Vitamins

Methylation is a biochemical process that is needed for all cells in the body. The process plays several key roles from providing cells with energy, to making and repairing DNA/RNA, and to eliminating toxins. It is important to understand and consider methylation because everyone has a different ability to methylate. Because of genetic polymorphisms or differences in genes that control methylation, some of us are better at it than others.

The problem is that methylation is needed for important metabolic processes such as making DNA and detoxifying chemicals. If methylation does not work well, serious health problems can ensue—such as heart disease, cancer, and autism, to name a few.

With genetic polymorphisms in methylation, some people cannot use the regular forms of folic acid and B12 (cyanocobalamin) found in most vitamins, including most prenatal vitamins. There are forms of these two vitamins that all people can use that are safe and effective. These are *folinic acid* or *methylfolate* for folic acid, and the *methylcobalamin form* (methyl B12) for vitamin B12. By giving women these forms directly we avoid problems from defects in methylation.

Benefits in children (relationship to autism)

The methylation process is vital to ensure a working detoxification system. Many children with autism have genetic polymorphisms that decrease their ability to methylate properly and therefore detoxify properly. This is compounded by a poor intake of nutrients (folic acid and vitamin B12) that are essential for methylation. Low nutrients before and during pregnancy can lead to low levels of nutrients in breast milk and, consequently, in breast-fed children.

Testing

A common test that is available is for *homocysteine*, a protein amino acid. Many doctors test it as a marker for heart disease. It should be a common test for women considering pregnancy because high levels of homocysteine are associated with negative pregnancy outcomes, including:

- Damage to the placenta, making it harder for nutrients to reach the baby[16]
- Increased risk of miscarriage[17]
- Preeclampsia (increase in the mother's blood pressure)[18]
- Birth defects (congenital heart disease, Down syndrome)

An ideal homocysteine level is ≤6 μmol/L, a moderately elevated level is considered 7 to 10 μmol/L; and a high level is >10 μmol/L. If the homocysteine level is high this means that methylation is not working as well as it should.

The homocysteine level in infants has been shown to correlate with their levels of folic acid and vitamin B12. The homocysteine level will increase without adequate intakes of these vitamins because the methylation pathways are blocked.

Another test that gives estimations of the levels of many B vitamins is called a *urine organic acid test*. If a local lab does this test, the results are normally to identify major genetic syndromes in metabolism. A related test is the *functional medicine organic acid test*. This gives estimates of B vitamin functions along with information on detoxification, mitochondria function, and even an imbalance of bacteria and yeast in the intestines. I routinely use this test for children with autism and find it very useful. Depending on a woman's health history, this test might also be very helpful.

Genetic tests can be done to determine genetic polymorphisms of the enzymes in the methylation pathway. By knowing if there are any specific enzyme genetic defects, a person can more directly target the nutrients needed. Because these tests are expensive, I do not routinely recommend them for women considering pregnancy. However, I do use these tests when caring for children with autism, especially if there is a strong family history of autism, a personal history of a previous child with autism, or recurrent pregnancy complications.

One enzyme that can be tested independently through a general laboratory is called the *MTHFR (methylenetetrahydrofolate reductase)* enzyme, which is critical in the methylation cycle. If there are polymorphisms in this enzyme it can lead to high homocysteine. Children with autism have an increased frequency of this polymorphism.

Supplementation before pregnancy

It makes sense that supplementing women before pregnancy can help prevent the development of autism in some children. Studies have shown that 400 mcg/day of methylation supplements is not enough to maintain supplement stores in breast milk.[19] Based on these studies, I recommend that all women considering pregnancy begin supplementing their diet with 1,000 mcg/day folinic acid and 1000 mcg/day methyl B12. If a woman has the MTHFR genetic polymorphism, I would consider taking another form of folate called L-5 methylfolate instead of the folinic acid. This is important if their homocysteine levels are not ≤ 6 µmol/L and especially important if the levels are >10 µmol/L. These vitamins are water-soluble and do not cause toxicity, as seen in some fat soluble vitamins such as vitamin A.

All prenatal vitamins contain folic acid and B12 but not all contain the correct forms. It is important to read the labels and look for folinic acid or methylfolate and methylcobalamin. If these forms were not present, then I would recommend an additional supplement of a multi-B complex vitamin with these forms. After beginning supplementation, I would then continue to check the homocysteine level until it reaches ≤6 µmol/L.

Table 6.2 - Laboratory Testing Summary

Mineral or vitamin	Laboratory test	Levels for a healthy pregnancy
Iron	Blood ferritin test	40 to 70 mcg/L
Zinc	RBC zinc	100 to 120 mcg/dL
Vitamin D	25-OH vitamin D level	50 to 80 ng/mL
Methylation vitamins	Homocysteine level	≤6 µmol/L

Abbreviations:
mcg/L = micrograms/liter; ng/mL = nanograms/milliliter;
µmol/L = micromoles/liter; ug/dL= micrograms/deciliter

Special Considerations for Vegetarians and Vegans

Vegetarians and vegans tend to have low levels of three important nutrients that exist primarily in animal products: iron, zinc, and vitamin B12. Women following these diets have special nutrition considerations when preparing their bodies for conception. Vegans do not eat animal or dairy products. Therefore, they are at the highest risk for deficiencies in these nutrients, calcium, and vitamin D. It is essential for vegetarian and vegan prospective parents to monitor their levels of these nutrients and to add supplements as needed to achieve proper nutrition levels.

Summary

Children with autism present with many nutritional deficits. Before pregnancy, women need to be tested for vitamin and mineral deficiencies and take supplements so that they have strong nutritional stores going into pregnancy. These high nutrition levels will help for better neurologic development in utero and the new child will start life with the building blocks they need to grow and develop normally.

CHAPTER 6 REFERENCES

1. Kaiser L, Allen LH, American Dietetic Association. Position of the American Dietetic Association: nutrition and lifestyle for a healthy pregnancy outcome. *J Am Diet Assoc.* 2008 Mar;108(3):553-61. DH468.

2. Schmidt RJ, Hansen RL, Hartiala J, Allayee H, Schmidt LC, Tancredi DJ, Tassone F, Hertz-Picciotto I. Prenatal vitamins, one-carbon metabolism gene variants, and risk for autism. *Epidemiology.* 2011 Jul;22(4):476-85. DH469.

3. Hellwig JP. Iron for infertility?: supplements appear protective. *Nurs Womens Health.* 2007 Feb;11(1):16-23. DH470.

4. Latif A, Heinz P, Cook R. Iron deficiency in autism and Asperger syndrome. *Autism.* Mar 2002: 6(1);103-114. DH471.

5. Cortese S, Azoulay R, Castellanos FX, Chalard F, Lecendreux M, Chechin D, Delorme R, Sebag G, Sbarbati A, Mouren MC, Bernardina BD, Konofal E. Brain iron levels in attention-deficit/hyperactivity disorder. A pilot MRI study. *World J Biol Psychiatry.* 2012 Mar;13(3):223-31. DH370.

6. Konofal E, Lecendreux M, Deron J, Marchand M, Cortese S, Zaïm M, Mouren MC. Arnulf I. Effects of iron supplementation on attention deficit hyperactivity disorder in children. *Pediatr Neurol.* 2008 Jan;38(1):20-6. DH375.

7. Beard JL. Why iron deficiency is important in infant development. *J Nutr.* 2008 Dec;138(12):2534-2536. DH193.

8. Eden AN, Sandoval C. Iron deficiency in infants and toddlers in the United States. *Pediatr Hematol Oncol.* 2012 Nov;29(8):704-9. DH472.

9. Scheplyagina LA. Impact of the mother's zinc deficiency on the woman's and newborn's health status. *J Trace Elem Med Biol.* 2005;19(1):29-35. DH325.

10. Caulfield LE, Zavaleta N, Shankar AH, Merialdi M. Potential contribution of maternal zinc supplementation during pregnancy to maternal and child survival. *Am J Clin Nutr.* 1998;68(suppl):499S-508S. DH322.

11. Gordon CM, Feldman HA, Sinclair L, Williams AL, Kleinman PK, Perez-Rossello J, Cox JE. Prevalence of vitamin D deficiency among healthy infants and toddlers. *Arch Pediatr Adoles Med. 2008* Jun;162(6):505-512. DH315.

12. Kočovská E, Fernell E, Billstedt E, Minnis H, Gillberg C. Vitamin D and autism: clinical review. *Res Dev Disabil.* 2012 Sep-Oct;33(5):1541-50. DH392.

13. Bener A, Alsaied A, Al-Ali M, Al-Kubaisi A, Basha B, Abraham A, Guiter G, Mian M. High prevalence of vitamin D deficiency in type 1 diabetes mellitus and healthy children. *Acta Diabetol.* 2008 Oct 10. DH312.

14. Bouwstra H, Dijck-Brouwer J, Decsi T, Boehm G, Boersma ER, Muskiet FA, Hadders-Algra M. Neurologic condition of healthy term infants at 18 months: positive association with venous umbilical DHA status and negative association with umbilical trans-fatty acids. *Pediatr Res.* 2006;60(3):334-339. DH31.

15. Dunstan JF, Simmer K, Dixon G, and Prescott SL. Cognitive assessment of children at age 2 ½ years after maternal fish oil supplementation in pregnancy: a randomized controlled trial. *Arch Dis Child Fetal Neonatal Ed.* 2008;93:F45-F50. DH32.

16. Bohles H, et. al. Maternal plasma homocysteine, placenta status and docosahexaenoic acid concentration in erythrocyte phospholipids of the newborn. *Eur J Pediatr.* 1999;158:243-246. DH11.

17. Govindaiah V, Naushad SM, Prabhakara K, Krishna PC, Radha Rama Devi A. Association of parental hyperhomocysteinemia and C677T methylene tetrahydrofolate reductase (MTHFR) polymorphism with recurrent pregnancy loss. *Clin Biochem.* 2009;42(4-5):380-386. DH12.

18. Kajdy A, Niemiec T. Homocysteine metabolism disorders as a potential predictor of preeclampsia. *Ginekol Pol.* 2008;79(11):775-779. DH16.

19. Molloy AM, Kirke PN, Brody LC, Scott JM, Mills JL. Effects of folate and vitamin B12 deficiencies during pregnancy on fetal, infant, and child development. *Food Nutr Bull.* 2008;29(2 Suppl):S101-11. DH532.

7

Building a Healthy Digestive System

A strong, well-functioning digestive system is essential for optimal health. It provides a vital link between good nutrition and the ability to detoxify harmful chemicals. The Triangle of Prevention points out the need for a woman to (1) eat healthy food and receive necessary nutrients, (2) have a functioning digestive system, and (3) avoid and remove toxins. If a woman's body is not able to absorb nutrients, it does not matter that she eats only organic whole foods. If her digestive system is not able to eliminate toxins, it does not matter that she tries to avoid toxins. Her body will just retain old toxins and acquire new ones that she cannot avoid.

This chapter describes common digestion problems and how to treat them effectively. The ideal time to do this is before pregnancy. Pregnancy will only exacerbate digestive ills such as constipation and heartburn.

Studies show that children with autism have more digestion problems than the general population.[1,2,3,4] Research has estimated that 70% of children with autism have some type of digestion problem.[5] There is a strong correlation of the severity of these symptoms with their severity of autism.[6] Indeed, most of the children I see in my practice with autism have digestive problems. Toward the end of this chapter, I describe a typical scenario of a two-year-old boy with both behavior issues and digestive problems. His digestion problems clearly affect his behavior. I illustrate how the digestion of the mother affects her child. Understanding the correlation between proper digestion and health is important for both the prevention and the treatment of autism.

Problems with digestion are extremely common in our population for multiple reasons:

- The current standard American diet (SAD) has high intakes of fast foods, soda, caffeine, and alcohol, but low intakes of vegetables and fiber.
- Processed and packaged foods contain chemical additives foreign to our digestive system.
- Antibiotics destroy the good bacteria in our intestines that lead to many digestive complaints. Antibiotics are common medicines and prevalent in our food supply.
- Our stressful lifestyles and eating on the run prevent us from relaxing—which is needed for proper digestion.

Common Digestion Problems

Some of the most common digestion problems a woman may have when preparing for pregnancy include:

Gastroesophageal reflux

Gastroesophageal reflux is also known as acid reflux or heartburn. It occurs when undigested food from the stomach comes back into the esophagus. This causes pain and burning. Medicines, such as Zantac™ and Prilosec™ are often taken to block stomach acid (hydrochloric acid or HCl) and reduce pain. They do not stop the actual reflux or the undigested food from coming into the esophagus. These medications treat only the symptoms, not the cause.

The use of these acid blockers can lead to digestive problems. Stomach acid is present for a reason: it is needed to break down proteins, kill infectious organisms in the stomach, and signal enzymes to be released. Insufficient acid impairs the proper breakdown and absorption of food.

Surprisingly, many people with reflux do not have enough stomach acid and actually have reflux symptoms caused by lack of acid instead of too much acid.

Irritable bowel

Symptoms caused by poor elimination, such as irritable bowel syndrome (IBS) and constipation, are common in both children and adults. IBS is a syndrome with alternating constipation/diarrhea, gas, bloating, and abdominal pain. According to traditional Western medicine, IBS has no "known" cause. People with IBS will often have a history of antibiotic use and have an imbalance between the good bacteria and other organisms in their gut.

Inflammatory Bowel Disease (IBD)

These colon disorders include Crohn's disease and ulcerative colitis. They are diagnosed by a blood test or biopsies of the intestine to detect inflammation, while a general diagnosis of IBS is based on symptoms.

Yeast imbalance

An imbalance of yeast or candida in the intestine can lead to symptoms such as irritable bowel syndrome, diarrhea, constipation, and bloating. It can also cause nonspecific signs and symptoms such as fatigue, headaches and vaginal yeast infections.

Bacteria imbalance

A severe imbalance of unwanted bacteria in the upper intestine is called *small bowel bacterial overgrowth*. This disorder can cause digestive symptoms and poor absorption of nutrients. It is also possible to have an imbalance of yeast and unwanted bacteria with a decreased amount of good bacteria or probiotics.

Elimination problems

Recurrent loose stools or diarrhea is another pattern of improper elimination. If diarrhea is persistent, a person can lose nutrients through their stools or be unable to absorb what they need from their food. Conversely, constipation can be a common problem. With constipation, the body retains waste (including toxins) for a longer period.

Constipation (due to our low-fiber standard American diet) is extremely common. It can cause symptoms such as pain, bloating, decreased appetite, and reduce a person's ability to detoxify.

Evaluation of Digestion

Fortunately there are good strategies to correct digestive problems: the causes can be identified with various tests and then effectively treated. Before pregnancy is a key time to detect and treat digestive issues. The resultant treatments will make pregnancy less symptomatic. They will also benefit the new child by giving the growing immune system, digestive system, and nutritional stores a necessary jump-start.

Digestive Tests

Some women are healthy and may not require digestive tests. However, depending on their symptoms and medical history, I recommend the following three tests (Table 7.1):

Complete digestive stool analysis (CDSA)

Usually, stool samples are tested for overt infections such as *salmonella* or *giardia*. A CDSA, however, can also check to see how well a person is digesting food and if there is a bacterial imbalance in the intestines. CDSA also shows the amounts of good bacteria (both lactobacillus and bifidus), the amounts of bacteria that are overgrown or should not be there at all, and if there is a possibility of overgrown yeast (often candida). The test also identifies if food is adequately being broken-down. If not, then we know there are problems with the amount of acid in the stomach and enzymes in the intestines. Enzymes aid digestion by breaking down proteins, fats, and carbohydrates from our food.

Urine organic acid test (OAT)

I order the urine OAT if I am concerned about an imbalance in the intestines due to either yeast or bad bacteria. These organisms release toxins in the form of acids, which are eliminated through urine.

Antibody protein (IgG) food allergy panel

Many digestive problems lead to a poor breakdown of proteins. As a result, it is common for people to have delayed food sensitivities or allergies created by an antibody protein (IgG) to specific foods. The IgG food allergy panel is a blood test that can identify these harmful reactions.

In addition to delayed food reactions created by IgG antibodies, people may react to foods in other ways. Immediate reactions to food, such as swelling of the throat are more obvious to people and often identified earlier in life. These will be detected by checking IgE food reactions, which can be done by most labs. Delayed reactions are more common and since the reactions do not happen directly after eating the food, correlation between food and symptom is difficult. Other parts of the immune system may cause food reactions and specialized tests are available that look at white blood cells and mast cells.

Table 7.1 - Recommended Digestive Tests

Test	Key findings	Reasons to order the test
Complete digestive stool analysis (CDSA)	- Good bacteria - Imbalanced bacteria - Imbalanced yeast - Enzymes - Inflammation	Antibiotic use, yeast infections, IBS, constipation, diarrhea, or inflammatory bowel disease
Urine organic acid test (OAT)	Elevated acids from yeast and bacteria	Antibiotic use, yeast infections, IBS, constipation, diarrhea, or inflammatory bowel disease
Antibody protein (IgG) food allergy panel	Elevated IgG levels for specific foods	Antibiotic use, yeast infections, IBS, constipation, diarrhea, inflammatory bowel disease, eczema, asthma, chronic congestion, runny nose, chronic headaches, or migraines

Probiotics

Probiotics are the good bacteria that live in our digestive system. Without them, people develop more problems with digestion, allergies, and infections. We first acquire good bacteria from our mother during birth and then nursing. As an adult, maintenance of these bacteria hap-

83

pens primarily through cultured food sources such as yogurt and kefir or supplements.

Unfortunately, most people do not have enough probiotic bacteria in their intestines. Modern manufactured foods lack these essential bacteria, and prescribed antibiotics kill both the bad and good bacteria. As a result, yeast and unwanted bacteria take over and create numerous digestive symptoms.

A woman before pregnancy should ensure that she has good gut flora in advance of pregnancy because they are very important for the start of her baby's health.

Probiotics during birth and nursing

Inside the uterus, infants have sterile intestines without bacteria. The infants need to ingest the mother's good bacteria to prime their own digestive and immune systems. Good bacteria that live in the intestines also live in the vaginal canal. This is important because infants normally travel head first through the canal during birth and ingest these bacteria into their own system. They also acquire good bacteria from nursing and close contact with their mothers.

Of course, babies born via cesarean section (C-section) do not travel down the vaginal canal and therefore do not receive good bacteria from the mother.[7,8,9] A higher percentage of children with autism and chronic digestive symptoms are born via C-section than children from the general population. Reasons for this increase are unclear. However, C-sections are sometimes necessary and can save the lives of both mothers and infants so should not be avoided if medically indicated. If a child is delivered by C-section, both the mother and infant need to begin probiotic supplementation.

Factors affecting maternal probiotics

Good bacteria cannot be passed along to the infant during birth and nursing if the mother does not have good bacteria during pregnancy or delivery. So it is important that a woman preparing for pregnancy begin to develop the needed probiotic flora. There are several reasons why a woman would lack good bacteria as she enters motherhood: (1) her body has an inadequate amount of probiotics, (2) an infection was treated with antibiotics, which destroy good bacteria, (3) she has a bacterial infection, or (4) there is a maternal imbalance of bacteria or yeast crowding out helpful bacteria.

Benefits of probiotics to newborns

It should be apparent by now that all women need one thing before pregnancy regardless of their medical history. That one thing is probiotics! A woman with adequate probiotics positively impacts the development of the infant's digestive and immune systems. Newborns need good bacteria right away. The time immediately following birth is a critical period for developing strong digestive and immune systems.[10,11]

Treatment of Digestion Problems

It is impossible to alleviate digestive problems when eating unhealthy food. Women cannot absorb nutrients from foods that do not have nutrients in the first place. Nutritious organic food is essential. Avoiding pesticides also means that the body does not have to work as hard to get rid of toxins. Table 7.2 lists recommended treatments for the disorders described below.

Reflux

Treatment for reflux involves decreasing heartburn pain and healing the lining of the esophagus and stomach. As stated, most medications prescribed for reflux may alleviate the symptoms, but the medicines also stop production of stomach acid, which is needed to break down proteins and assist digestion.

Alternative treatment options (such as colostrum, the amino acid glutamine, deglycerized licorice, and aloe vera) decrease the symptoms of reflux without stopping stomach acid. They also decrease inflammation so the digestive tract can heal.

To effectively reduce reflux, women often need to make dietary changes, slow down their eating, and use other digestive support such as probiotics and the alternative treatments listed above.

Irritable Bowel Syndrome

The symptoms of IBS often resolve when the imbalance of bacteria and yeast is corrected (known as dysbiosis treatment). Diarrhea may be handled in the same way. For many digestive complaints like IBS, the problem is that the food is not being broken-down properly. Adding enzymes and sometimes stomach acid (HCl) may help. The digestive stool test can identify problems with food breakdown before or during supplement replacement. However, sometimes treatment can be empiric, meaning that different treatments need to be tried before finding a solution to the problem.

Bacterial infection

I usually first treat the bacterial imbalance with probiotics and herbs such as grapefruit seed extract, caprylic acid, or garlic. If the combination of probiotics and herbs is ineffective, antibiotics may also be prescribed. However, it is imperative to prevent yeast overgrowth during antibiotic treatment.

Yeast Imbalance

A yeast imbalance is treated with high doses of probiotics in addition to one or more or the above-mentioned herbs. An anti-yeast prescription medicine may also be given. Because sugar causes yeast to grow, it is also important for a woman to decrease her sugar intake including concentrated fruit sugar in processed juices.

Elimination

The cause of an elimination problem must first be identified before appropriate treatment can be started.

For diarrhea the first step is to determine if one or more foods are contributing to the symptoms. This can be a food that is an allergen or foods that when eaten in excess lead to diarrhea such as excessive fruit juice. Probiotics are essential and I often recommend adding the probiotic S Boulardii for diarrhea.

If constipation is an issue, a goal is to have at least one stool per day. Adding more fruit, vegetables, fiber, nutritional oils (olive, coconut, or cod liver oil), and water to the diet are important first steps.

I often recommend additional nutrients to help relieve constipation. Magnesium is a mineral that causes relaxation of the smooth muscle including the intestines. The levels of magnesium in the body are inversely proportional to the levels of calcium. Because calcium is more common in the Western diet, our magnesium levels are often low. Milk of Magnesia is a common over-the-counter treatment for constipation and can be a very effective treatment. The main problem with Milk of Magnesia is that it does not contain the most absorbable form of magnesium. Magnesium glycinate, magnesium citrate, and ionic magnesium are better absorbable forms to help nutrient stores and constipation. Too much magnesium leads to diarrhea, and reducing the level before loose stools begin is a good estimate of how much magnesium the body needs.

Vitamin C in high doses can also get the bowels moving. Our bodies need vitamin C, and it is considered very safe. Similar to magnesium, too much vitamin C may cause diarrhea. And again, probiotics will help the intestines.

Table 7.2 - Recommended Treatments for Digestion Problems

Treatment	Recommended treatment options	Recommended amounts
Stomach acid (HCl)*	Treatment options (use only one): Betaine HCl Raw apple cider vinegar Swedish bitters Gentian root extract	With each meal: 1 capsule ½ t ½ t 100 mg

Probiotics: Combination of several lactobacillus and bifidus strains	Commercial probiotic brands. Cultured foods: kefir and kombucha	Daily recommendations:
		Initial:
		  5 billion CFU
		Maintenance:
		  20 billion CFU
		Treatment:
		  100 billion+ CFU

Healthy organic food	All healthy organic food	Maintain a healthy weight
Regular elimination	Healthy diet, fiber, nutritional oils, water, Magnesium citrate or glycinate Vitamin C	 200-600 mg daily 1,000 mg daily
Digestive enzymes*	Commercially available brands	With each meal: 1-2 capsules
Healing the intestine*	Treatment options (use at least one or as needed): Colostrum Glutamine Deglycerized licorice Aloe vera	Daily recommendations: 500-3,000 mg 1,000-3,000 mg 500-1,500 mg Juice: 2-8 oz or capsules

*Not all women/children will need these treatments

Note: CFU = colony-forming units

Clinical Example: Jonathan, Age 2

The following case illustrates a pattern that I see frequently in children with autism and digestive problems. You will see that the mother-child health link is strong and that the mother's digestive status, both at the onset of and throughout pregnancy, has a very large influence on her baby's digestion and overall health.

A woman came into my practice with her 2-year-old son.

"Jonathan hasn't gained weight in 6 months," the mother told me. "He has this terrible diarrhea every day and always seems cranky. My son's first doctor said he has toddler's diarrhea and not to worry about it. But Jonathan isn't getting better, and now I am worried because he isn't growing anymore. I have also noticed his behavior is getting worse with more temper tantrums and acting out."

I asked more about Jonathan's birth and how he was fed as a baby. According to the mother, he had a normal birth and was a good "nurser" for the first year of life. When asked further if he was a fussy baby, she said, "Well, he was colicky, and he did spit up his food a lot. His doctor said it was reflux and gave him some medicine for it. It didn't help very much, so I stopped it."

I then asked whether Jonathan had a lot of infections and was taking any medicines. "After he was one year old and stopped nursing, he started to get ear infections all the time. He was put on antibiotics, but he never seemed to get better. After that, he started getting diarrhea and being fussy. Now every time I take him to the doctor, he never seems to gain any weight."

There is a strong connection between the health of a mother and child, so I began asking the mother about her health. "I have no medical problems—or nothing serious." When asked if she had ever taken medications, the mother replied, "Well, I did take antibiotics for acne several years ago. And when I was working, I was really stressed and had heartburn. So I had some medicine for that, which helped the pain."

I asked about her pregnancy and whether she was sick at all. "I did have some yeast infections, but doesn't every pregnant woman? I also had some bacteria that they found right before the baby was born."

"Was that group B strep?" I asked.

"That sounds right. They gave me some medicine in an IV during delivery to get rid of it, some type of antibiotic I think."

This example demonstrates a chain of events that began with the mother and was unknowingly passed down to her infant. Because the mother was treated with long-term antibiotics for acne, the good bacteria in her intestines were destroyed. This led to vaginal yeast infections, a sign that she also had an overgrowth of yeast in the intestines. The reflux was treated with an acid blocker even though the mom may have actually had insufficient stomach acid. At delivery, the IV antibiotics further destroyed any good bacteria in the mother's body. So Jonathan did not receive any good bacteria during birth or during nursing.

Without good bacteria, Jonathan was not able to digest his food well. Most likely he had pain, which led to colic and reflux. The reflux was treated with an acid blocker, which limited his ability to break down proteins, resulting in further pain and discomfort. Jonathan's body then began to react to unbroken-down proteins. This caused delayed food reactions, especially following the introduction of a large quantity of dairy products. The delayed food reaction to dairy, in turn, caused chronic nose congestion, leading to fluid in the ears and frequent ear infections. Antibiotics were given for these ear infections, which destroyed some of his good bacteria. A resulting overgrowth of bad bacteria and yeast caused diarrhea. These bacteria and yeast released toxins and caused pain leading to behavior issues such as temper tantrums.

Although this is a complicated history, I see similar scenarios frequently. It is easy to see how one thing leads to another. If the mother had a good intake of probiotics before, during, and after pregnancy and if Jonathan was given probiotics after birth, a lot of these problems could have been avoided. Even a simple intervention of probiotics can lead to a substantial decrease in a chain of significant health problems.

Summary

Hopefully, it is clear that good digestion is important for good health. Sometimes improving health can be as easy as supplementing with good probiotic bacteria or even adding more cultured foods into the diet. For chronic digestion problems it is vital to consult with a trained health care provider.

There is a strong link between the mother's and baby's digestive health. Understanding that digestion and behavior are connected is critical for both the treatment and the prevention of autism. In my practice, I rarely have a child with autism that I do not need to treat for digestive problems. And with treatment, they feel and act better. I am convinced that better digestion in mothers-to-be and babies will help prevent autism.

CHAPTER 7 REFERENCES

1. Adams JB, Johansen L, Powell L, Quig D, Rubin R. Gastrointestinal flora and gastrointestinal status in children with autism -- comparisons to typical children and correlation with autism severity. *BMC Gastroenterol.* 2011;11:22. DH380.

2. Horvath K, Perman JA. Autistic disorder and gastrointestinal disease. *Curr Opin Pediatr.* 2002;14(5):583-587. DH69.

3. Buie T, et al. Evaluation, diagnosis and treatment of gastrointestinal disorders in individuals with ASDs: a consensus report. *Pediatrics.* 2010;125(suppl 1):S1-S18. DH56.

4. Parracho HM, Bingham MO, Gibson GR, McCartney AL. Differences between the gut microflora of children with autistic spectrum disorders and that of healthy children. *J Med Microbiol.* 2005;54(pt 10):987-991. DH77.

5. Coury DL, Ashwood P, Fasano A, Fuchs G, Geraghty M, Kaul A, Mawe G, Patterson P, Jones N. Gastrointestinal conditions in children with autism spectrum disorder: developing a research agenda. *Pediatrics.* 2012 Nov: 130;S160-8. DH531.

6. Adams 2011.

7. Grönlund MM, Lehtonen OP, Eerola E, Kero P. Fecal microflora in healthy infants born by different methods of delivery: permanent changes in intestinal flora after cesarean delivery. *J Pediatr Gastroenterol Nutr.* 1999;28(1):19-25. DH65.

8. Biasucci G, Benenati B, Morelli L, Bessi E, Boehm G. Cesarean delivery may affect the early biodiversity of intestinal bacteria. *J Nutr.* 2008;138(9):1796S-1800S. DH55.

9. Penders J, et al. Factors influencing the composition of the intestinal microbiota in early infancy. *Pediatrics.* 2006;118(2):511-512. DH78.

10. Conroy ME, Shi HN, Walker WA. The long-term health effects of neonatal microbial flora. *Curr Opin Allergy Clin Immunol.* 2009;9(3):197-201. DH58.

11. Morelli L. Postnatal development of intestinal microflora as influenced by infant nutrition. *J Nutr.* 2008;138(9):1791S-1795S. DH73.

8

Strengthening the Immune System

Inflammation is the immune system's response to something foreign to the body. It is the underlying problem in many chronic diseases including autism. In children with autism, inflammation is present in the brain[1] and the intestines[2] and probably other organs as well. The causes of this inflammation are unclear but it does appear that in some children with autism, their mothers have evidence of immune problems and autoimmune disease[3] (when the body attacks its own healthy tissue). The mother has immune antibodies towards the fetus.[4,5,6] If a woman has a fever or gets the flu (influenza) during pregnancy, her child is more likely to develop autism.[7] The flu infection, or the immune response to the infection, in the mother signals the fetus to mount an inflammatory response. Inflammation in the mother from any cause is associated with an increase in autism in her children.

Therefore, it follows that if women can strengthen their immune systems before pregnancy, they will have less risk of inflammation and infections with less risk of passing infections and abnormal antibodies to their infants.

Immune System Problems

There are three categories of problems that arise from a poorly functioning immune system: (1) immunodeficiencies, (2) autoimmunity, and (3) hypersensitivity (including allergic reactions). These are all becoming more common.

Immunodeficiency is the term used to describe an immune system that is unable to respond adequately to an infection, causing a person to get sick more quickly or more frequently. Immunodeficiency can be from a disease a person is born with or it can be acquired, such as the Human Immunodeficiency Virus (HIV). Our lifestyle can also lead to poor immune function. General malnutrition, inadequate protein, and specific deficiencies in iron, zinc, selenium, vitamins A, C, E, D, B6, and folic acid can all lead to weaker immune function. Stress depresses immune function. Most people realize they get more colds when they are stressed and run down.

Autoimmunity is when the immune system misidentifies normal cells as foreign and mounts an immune system response against these healthy tissues. The immune system can attack thyroid cells in Hashimoto's thyroiditis, or cells in joints in rheumatoid arthritis. In type 1 diabetes, the pancreas is attacked, and in multiple sclerosis (MS) brain cells are attacked. *Celiac disease* is the autoimmune reaction to glutenous grains in the diet, which then cause attack on the lining of the intestine.

Hypersensitivity reactions or allergy reactions are when the immune system causes damages to tissues. The damaged tissues lead to the symptoms common in allergies. Common allergic reactions include hay fever or seasonal allergies, hives, food reactions, some types of asthma, and eczema. Some reactions are immediate and mediated by antibodies called *Immunoglobulin E* or IgE (an example would be a life-threatening reaction that happens in certain people to peanuts where their throat closes up). Other antibodies, such as IgG, IgM, and IgA can cause more delayed reactions as seen with reactions to foods.

Immune System Problems in Autism

Children with autism have many well-documented problems with their immune systems,[8,9] including the problems described above. These children have deficiencies in their immune systems leading to increased infections.[10] They have decreased numbers of, and poorly functioning, natural killer cells that lead to problems fighting viruses.[11] Their white blood cells produce less disease fighting antibodies leading to increased infections.

Autoimmune reactions are also common in children with autism.[12] Antibodies against their brains' proteins have been found in blood tests showing elevated myelin basic proteins and neurofilament proteins.[13,14] These elevated proteins show that inflammation is occurring in their brains. The inflammation presents with head pain and difficulty thinking, speaking, and processing. Research has shown a correlation between certain viral infections and elevated antibodies in the mother to fetal brain tissue.[15,16] Autoimmune diseases are also more common in the mothers and other family members of those children with autism.[17,18] Multiple types of allergies are common in children with autism and include reactions such as asthma, eczema, seasonal allergies, and multiple reactions to foods. These can be life-threatening reactions to foods or delayed reactions with nasal congestion, spaciness, and bloating from eating a specific food.

Infections in Autism

Because of immune problems, infections are seen more commonly in children with autism.[19] Many of these children have recurrent ear infections or respiratory infections. These children not only have recurrent illnesses, but also take longer to recover from them than other children. The immune systems of these children overreact to some infections. When we analyze their blood, we often find high levels of antibodies (indicating a continuing fight with a pathogen) and ongoing inflammation.

Infectious viruses that have been studied include herpes 6 (seen with the common childhood disorder roseola) and other herpes infections. Case studies have shown that when a person gets a herpes-induced infection in the brain called *encephalitis* they develop symptoms similar to autism.[20] Upon treatment, the symptoms can be reversed. Researchers are reviewing responses to other viruses. For example, some children respond to the measles virus with very high antibodies and they improve with anti-viral treatment.

Bacterial infections such as recurrent strep infections or bladder infections are common in children with autism. In some children, the strep bacteria lead to the development of an autoimmune reaction which is known as *Pediatric Autoimmune Disease Associated with Strep (PANDAS)*. Children afflicted with PANDAS often exhibit rage, obsessive compulsive disorders and, less often, tics. Children can have problems with skin infections from *methicillin resistant staph aureus (MRSA)*.

Overgrowth of yeast (often candida) and harmful bacteria in the intestines is very common in these children and contributes frequently to the digestive symptoms in children with autism. Intestinal parasites often coexist with yeast and bacteria in the intestine.

Correlation Between Immune System Disorders in Autism and Prevention

Since we know that there are immune system problems in children with autism, we need to determine how these immune problems developed and how to prevent these problems from happening in the first place. Probiotics and the development of the digestive system (which is integral to the immune system) play a critically important role. A child who receives good bacteria from their mother has the first step toward developing a healthy immune system. Since there are many ways the proper transfer of good bacteria to the baby can be disrupted (C-section, maternal antibiotics, infant antibiotics, or lack of breast feeding), probiotic supplementation of both the mother and the infant is a good next step.

Correlation Between Prenatal Infections and Autism

It has been known for decades that if a mother is exposed to certain viruses during pregnancy that there is an increased risk of developmental problems in the infant.

Exposure to rubella during pregnancy is a known risk factor for the development of autism.[21] Rubella is not very common anymore and women are screened for antibodies to rubella when they are pregnant. If a woman is not immune, it is recommended that she be vaccinated immediately after pregnancy. Since rubella is a live virus vaccine, I have concerns about giving a nursing mother this vaccine. If the woman is nursing she will pass antibodies to her child, which may have negative effects on an infant's immune system in a similar manner to a woman who is pregnant and exposed to rubella. The vaccine will alter her immune system and the baby's immune system and isn't worth the risk since we know rubella can lead to the development of autism. We should be careful and not potentially expose an infant through breast milk when we do not know the full impact of that decision and the risk of rubella infection is low.

Rubella is part of a group of infections called *TORCH*. These infections include Toxoplasmosis, Other (includes hepatitis B, coxsackie viruses, syphilis, chickenpox, HIV, parvovirus B12-Fifth disease), Rubella, Cytomegalovirus, and Herpes. These infections can lead to problems in the newborn from congenital birth defects to developmental delay. The TORCH infections commonly affect the heart, skin, eyes, and nervous system. The most common problems seen include *chorioretinitis* or inflammation in the eye, *microcephaly* which is a small head, and *focal cerebral calcifications* which are calcium deposits in the brain. Depending on the stage during pregnancy of exposure, afflicted infants can also be born small for their age, have rashes, enlarged liver/kidneys, jaundice, problems with hearing, mental retardation, and autism. The mothers during pregnancy often show no signs of infection or only mild symptoms.

Most obstetricians screen for these infections during pregnancy. If identified during pregnancy, both toxoplasmosis and syphilis can be treated with antibiotics. If rubella or chickenpox screens don't show a woman is immune, obstetricians may offer vaccines but I believe it is generally better to wait until after pregnancy and nursing for any immunizations because of potential immune risks to the infant, which we do not yet fully understand.

Prevention of these infections is different depending on the infection. Toxoplasmosis is common in cats, and pregnant woman are told not to change the cat's litter box specifically to prevent exposure. Syphilis, HIV, and herpes are sexually transmitted so safe sex is key. Hepatitis B can be transmitted by sex or by IV drug use, so again, prevention is possible. Some of the other infections are more common in children, such as chickenpox, parvovirus, and herpes 6 (roseola). It is important for pregnant women to avoid contact with sick children as much as possible. Obviously for pediatricians, teachers, and mothers this is difficult to do. Many people who have worked with children for many years have already been exposed and have immunity. The chief concern is having first time exposure during pregnancy that causes an acute inflammatory response in the mother and causes infection and inflammation in the fetus.

Overall, the best way of preventing infections is for the mother to avoid exposures and to have a strong immune system before getting pregnant, during pregnancy, and early childhood. This will allow her to pass along a strong immune system to her new baby.

Correlation Between Autism and Maternal Antibodies

Recent troubling research has shown that a subset of mothers who have children with autism had developed antibodies during pregnancy that attacked the brain of the fetus.[22] We know that protective antibodies cross into the placenta from the mother; however, it appears that harmful antibodies can cross into the placenta too. These autoantibodies can cause temporary problems, such as the case of myasthenia gravis or longer lasting problems as seen with lupus. At this time it is unclear why a woman would develop antibodies to her own child's brain, but a woman with autoimmune issues or an over reactive immune system with many allergies is more likely to have children with these problems.

Strengthening the Immune System

Since there are three ways in which the immune system causes problems [(1) immunodeficiencies, (2) autoimmunity, and (3) hypersensitivity], it is important to address each area in order to have a strong and balanced immune system. A woman preparing for pregnancy should build up a weakened immune system, treat any ongoing infections, and decrease an overactive immune system from having autoimmune or allergic reactions. All of these approaches lead to a final goal of decreasing inflammation, which is the underlying problem in all chronic diseases, including infections, autoimmune diseases, allergies, autism, and heart disease. Depending on the chronicity of problems, this can take a long time to do. Again, the best time to do immune strengthening is before becoming pregnant.

Identification and treatment of a weakened immune system

Most people know if they have a weakened immune system. They seem to get infections more easily and it takes them longer to recover than other people. Usually building up a weak immune system can be done through basic self-care. Decreasing stress and increasing sleep help to build a stronger immune system. Dietary changes such as increasing fruits/vegetables and adequate protein are important. Since sugar depresses immunity, decreasing sugar and simple carbohydrates is important. I can always tell when flu and cold season begins because it correlates to the holidays when people start eating a lot of sugar (beginning with Halloween).

If a woman is getting sick frequently, I recommend extra nutrients to help the immune system. These include vitamin D (especially in the winter to achieve a blood level of 50). She should take extra vitamin C; it is a water soluble vitamin and is very safe. Extra zinc is also good since most people are low in this nutrient. These recommendations are part of a general healthy diet and supplement regimen as described in previous chapters. When women are building healthy eating habits and nutrient stores, they are also building a strong immune system.

If someone has done the above steps and is still getting sick frequently, I often have them take herbs to help build the immune system. There are individual herbs such as astragalus, which is given in capsules or tincture twice daily. These are good treatments for respiratory infections but are not to be given during acute illnesses or fevers. Echinacea is helpful for short (often two-week) courses to build immunity. Elderberry works well for preventing or treating influenza-type illnesses. Many companies offer herbal immune-building formulas. Immune-building formulas also exist that contain herbs and glandulars such as thymus. If a woman needs the strength of glandulars, it is wise to work with a knowledgeable health care practitioner.

When the adrenal glands are weak, people often have problems resisting infections. The next chapter will describe adrenal function, weakness, and remedies. In our stressful society, having weak adrenals and being "burned out" is quite common, and leads to many immune system problems.

Another supplement to boost the immune system is cow-derived colostrum. Colostrum helps build immunity through supportive antibodies and is especially good for healing the intestine. There are also formulas that isolate the protective antibodies for even further strengthening. For weak responses to viruses or low levels of natural killer cells, which can result in weaker responses to viruses, transfer factors are very helpful. They literally "transfer immunity" to a person who does not have good immunity themselves. Health care providers often recommend IgG and transfer factor products.

Summary for strengthening immune system

1. Stress reduction
2. Adequate rest and sleep
3. Decreasing sugars and simple carbohydrates
4. Increasing fruits and vegetables
5. Adequate protein to make antibodies
6. Extra vitamin C and D
7. Extra zinc and selenium
8. Herbal support: individual astragalus, elderberry, or combination products
9. Colostrum or oral antibody supplements
10. Identification and treatment of weak adrenal glands (next chapter)

Identification and Treatment of Infections

It is important to identify and treat any infections before pregnancy, especially any chronic infections. I already discussed a common type of infection that exists in the intestine, which is an imbalance of bacteria and yeast called dysbiosis. Since this imbalance can be passed onto a child, it is important to treat before pregnancy and definitely before delivery.

Vaginal infections need to be addressed for similar reasons since the imbalanced bacteria can be passed to the newborn infant. It is common for women to have vaginal yeast infections and this can directly lead to digestive problems, thrush, colic, and diaper rash in a newborn infant—not to mention the chronic digestion problems often seen in children with autism.

Chronic sinus infections can produce an overgrowth of yeast if they have been treated repeatedly with antibiotics. Again the treatment for all of these issues above is high doses of probiotics, lower sugar in the diet, and herbal anti-fungals. Sometimes prescription anti-fungals may be needed if the previous treatments are not effective.

Some people harbor chronic infections such as herpes. Herpes is an infection that tends to stay with people throughout their lives. It is important to keep the infection controlled. Stress usually can bring on an acute herpes outbreak, either oral or vaginal. A common amino acid called *lysine* helps to keep the herpes virus at bay. Natural anti-virals such as monolaurin can be helpful along with general immune support listed above. Prescription anti-virals can also be useful.

Lyme Disease and Chronic Fatigue Syndrome

An organization called the *Lyme Induced Autism Foundation* (www.lymeinducedautism.com) has extensive information on Lyme disease, especially chronic Lyme disease and its myriad of symptoms. Serious concern has been raised about prenatal transmission of Lyme disease and its role in the development of autism. If a woman has chronic fatigue and multiple medical complaints that have not been addressed, she should be evaluated by an integrative health care practitioner to test for Lyme and other chronic infections and treated properly before attempting to get pregnant. These are serious infections and difficult to treat. Treatment often involves not only antibiotics but also treatment of hormone problems and allergies.

Identification and Treatment of Allergies

Most people know if they have acute allergies to foods, or seasonal allergies such as hay fever. If they have multiple non-specific symptoms such as chronic congestion, headaches, stomach pain, bloating, gassiness, irritable bowel symptoms, wheezing, or eczema they should look for delayed allergies or sensitivities to foods. A diet that eliminates the most allergenic foods for at least two weeks often gives information on food reactions. Once all the symptoms disappear, foods should be introduced one at a time until the symptoms come back. If the elimination diet isn't helpful and there is still concern about food reactions, a delayed food reaction panel test can be ordered. The way to get rid of a food reaction is to remove the food. For delayed food reactions, the removal may only have to be for 6 months in order for the inflammation to decrease and the immune system to calm down.

One of the best things to help decrease allergies—as you might guess—is probiotics. Yes, these bacteria in our intestines help modify allergic reactions. They are very helpful even for skin reactions such as eczema.

Vitamin C and quercetin are two other supplements that are natural anti-histamines and good for treating allergies. Vitamin C is helpful for fighting infections and fighting allergies. Again, a higher dose vitamin C is needed. Quercetin is a phytonutrient in that it naturally exists in plants, such as pink fruits. Doses of 1000 mg a day are often needed to help decrease allergy symptoms, and often come together with vitamin C, again in 1000 mg doses.

Stinging nettles is an herb that is good for allergies and can be found in products with vitamin C and quercetin. Homeopathic formulas and Chinese herbal formulas specifically designed for allergies are also available.

For women with multiple chronic allergies, immunotherapy by an integrated medical provider or allergist is an option. The therapy can be via oral/sublingual or allergy shots.

Identification and Treatment of Inflammation

Inflammation is the end result of any immune system activation or infection. It is ultimately what causes the symptoms of infection or autoimmune reactions. It is present in all chronic diseases, including autism. Strengthening the immune system also means decreasing inflammation.

Prescription medicines are available that decrease inflammation. Unfortunately they have side effects that make long-term use unsafe. The most common medicines are called *NSAIDs* or *non-steroidal anti-inflammatory drugs such as ibuprofen*. Steroids are also anti-inflammatory and are used to treat many diseases, especially chronic autoimmune diseases. Steroids are good in acute situations if medically necessary but carry serious long-term side effects. Ibuprofen use can also have long-term consequences. It is metabolized in the kidneys and can be of concern to those with chronic kidney problems. It can also cause bleeding in the intestine, which can be life-threatening if severe.

Luckily, there are many natural anti-inflammatory foods and supplements. An anti-inflammatory diet includes lots of natural antioxidants, which work to decrease inflammation. These anti-oxidants are high in all fruits and vegetables. Multiple vegetables and fruits can decrease inflammation on a daily basis. However, many saturated fats in meats and dairy products tend to be pro-inflammatory.

For supplements, omega-3 fish oils in cod liver oil or fish oil are anti-inflammatory. They help the immune system, decrease heart disease, help prevent depression, and, for a baby, improve brain development. Probiotics have an anti-inflammatory effect by helping balance the immune system.

There are also individual herbs and combination products that decrease inflammation. One of my favorites is an Indian spice called *curcumin* or *turmeric*. It needs to be taken with a source of fat in the diet or in a more absorbable form. There are combination products specifically formulated to decrease pain by decreasing inflammation. Products targeted for chronic joint pain often also contain many natural anti-inflammatory agents. Several of the detoxification formulas in later chapters have multiple anti-inflammatory supplements in them.

Summary

Inflammation is an underlying factor in disease, especially chronic diseases such as autism. Preventing inflammation in the child is therefore integral to preventing autism in the child. Since we know that problems in the mother's immune system can cause problems in the infant, we have to treat the mother first before pregnancy. Decreasing her inflammation and balancing her immune system are critical for her health and her child's health. We have a lot to learn about the immune system's interrelationship between mother and child, but we can make a big difference in the health of the child with what we now know.

CHAPTER 8 REFERENCES

1. Vargas DL, Nascimbene C, Krishnan C, Zimmerman AW, Pardo CA. Neuroglial activation and neuroinflammation in the brain of patients with autism. *Ann Neurol.* 2005:57(1):67-81. DH87.

2. Horvath K, Perman JA. Autism and gastrointestinal symptoms. *Curr Gastroenterol Rep.* 2002;4(3):251-258. DH68.

3. Brown SA, Sourander A, Hinkka-Yli-Salomäki S, McKeague IW, Sundvall J, Surcel H-M. Elevated maternal C-reactive protein and autism in a national birth cohort. *Mol Psychiatry.* 2013 Jan 22. DH568.

4. Comi AM, Zimmerman AW, Frye VH, Law PA, Peeden JN. Familial clustering of autoimmune disorders and evaluation of medical risk factors in autism. *J Child Neurol.* 1999. June;14(6):388-94. DH146.

5. Enstrom AM, Van de Water JA, Ashwood P. Autoimmunity in autism. *Curr Opin Investig Drugs.* 2009 May;10(5):463-73. DH365.

6. Fox E, Amaral D, Van de Water J. Maternal and fetal antibrain antibodies in development and disease. *Dev Neurobiol.* 2012 Oct;72(10):1327-34. DH408.

7. Atladóttir HÓ, Henriksen TB, Schendel DE, Parner ET. Autism after infection, febrile episodes, and antibiotic use during pregnancy: an exploratory study. *Pediatrics.* 2012 Dec;130(6):e1447-54. DH474.

8. Comi 1999.

9. Cohly HH, Panja A. Immunological findings in autism. *Int Rev Neurobiol.* 2005;71:317. DH362.

10. Comi 1999.

11. Ashwood P, Krakowiak P, Hertz-Picciotto I, Hansen R, Pessah IN, Van de Water J. Altered T cell responses in children with autism. *Brain Behav Immun.* 2011 Jul;25(5):840-9. DH344.

12. Atladottir HO, et al. Association of family history of autoimmune diseases and autism spectrum disorders. *Pediatrics.* 2009 Aug;124(2):687-94. DH146.

13. Singh VK, Warren RP, Odell JD, Warren WL, Cole P. Antibodies to myelin basic protein in children with autistic behavior. *Brain Behav Immun.* 1993 Mar;7(1):97-103. DH478.

14. Connolly AM, Chez M, Streif EM, Keeling RM, Golumbek PT, Kwon JM, Riviello JJ, Robinson RG, Neuman RJ, Deuel RM. Brain-derived neurotrophic factor and autoantibodies to neural antigens in sera of children with autistic

spectrum disorders, Landau-Kleffner syndrome, and epilepsy. *Biol Psychiatry.* 2006 Feb 15;59(4):354-63. DH477.

15. Enstrom 2009.

16. Fox 2012.

17. Atladottir HO, et al. Association of family history of autoimmune diseases and autism spectrum disorders. *Pediatrics.* 2009 Aug;124(2):687-94. DH145.

18. Comi 1999.

19. Konstantareas MM, Homatidis S. Ear infections in autistic and normal children. *J Autism Dev Disord.* 1987 Dec;17(4):585-94. DH476.

20. Ghaziuddin M, Al-Khouri I, Ghaziuddin N. Autistic symptoms following herpes encephalitis. *Eur Child Adolesc Psychiatry.* 2002 Jun;11(3):142-6. DH475.

21. Patterson PH. Maternal infection and immune involvement in autism. *Trends Mol Med.* 2011 Jul;17(7):389-94. DH361.

22. Elovitz MA, Brown AG, Breen K, Anton L, Maubert M, Burd I. Intrauterine inflammation, insufficient to induce parturition, still evokes fetal and neonatal brain injury. *Int J Dev Neurosci.* 2011 Oct;29(6):663-71. DH363.

9

Hormones: The Balancing Act

Hormones are our body's chemical messengers. They are produced in certain glands, such as the thyroid, and sent through the body as signals to control metabolism and reproduction. Hormones keep the body functioning smoothly.

With hormones, balance is key. If hormones levels are too high or too low, they can affect the entire body. Hormones are also interrelated, so an imbalance of adrenal hormones may put stress on the thyroid. Having an imbalance in thyroid hormones often affects the steroid hormones, estrogen and progesterone, and leads to problems with fertility.

Unfortunately, today we have external factors that can shift our hormones in unhealthy directions. Any stress felt in our bodies from our environment, whether it is emotional or physical, will cause a release extra hormones to try to combat the stress. The hormone system was designed for responding to acute stress, such as being chased by a wild animal. Luckily today we are not often faced with this scenario, but having ongoing day-to-day stress can lead our body to believe we are in a constant fight for our lives. Eventually, chronic stress takes a toll on our hormonal system, leading to imbalances that can affect every function in the body.

Today, there are also many chemicals, from plastics to ingredients in cosmetics that mimic hormones in the body. Many of these act as estrogen or thyroid hormones. It is easy to imagine how an outside chemical that acts like estrogen in the body could affect a woman's ability to become pregnant. For a pregnant woman, every chemical that circulates in her body will travel through the placenta to the baby. It is frightening to me that a pregnant woman could be exposed to a chemical that could affect not only her hormones to maintain a pregnancy, but also the hormones of her unborn child.

This chapter provides a basic review of hormones. With this knowledge we can see that all of the hormones, not just estrogen and progesterone, are involved in fertility, maintaining a healthy pregnancy, and having a healthy child. Balancing these hormones before pregnancy is a key factor in achieving these goals.

Stress and Pregnancy Outcome

Stress during pregnancy can have negative effects on the baby, including preterm delivery and low birth weight.[1] In addition to physical problems, stress can lead to poor development of the nervous system. One animal study showed that stress during pregnancy had long lasting negative effects on the neurodevelopment of offspring.[2] Another study reviewed the relation of maternal stress to autism and found that stress can disrupt normal fetal neurologic development, leading to an increased risk of autism.[3] Stress may also play a role in gene-environment interactions or epigenetic changes.[4]

I know from personal experience how stress can negatively affect pregnancy and the health of a new baby. When I was pregnant with my second child, I was a pediatrician in a busy practice with an active two year old at home, a busy husband, and the possibility of a move to a new state in the near future. Halfway through my pregnancy I began to have contractions and became concerned that I was going into preterm labor. As my stress and the pregnancy continued, my daughter's growth slowed down. Eventually the doctors said her growth had stopped, her delivery was induced and she was born over three weeks early. The placenta was noted to be small but they couldn't find any cause. I knew it was because of stress. She then went on to be a colicky baby who cried all the time and had difficulty gaining weight. There was no question in my mind that stress had a profound effect not only on my health, but the health of my baby.

Types of Hormones

Although there are many hormones in the body, I will focus on three main groups of hormones that are important for a healthy pregnancy and a healthy child: (1) the adrenal hormones, (2) the thyroid hormones, and (3) the steroid hormones (estrogen and progesterone). We will cover the basic functions of these hormones and what symptoms would indicate an imbalance.

Adrenal Hormones

The adrenal glands are located on top of the kidneys. They consist of two parts: the outer part called the *cortex,* and the inner part called the *medulla.*

The adrenal cortex produces 3 types of steroid hormones, all of which are essential for life. The first is *aldosterone,* which is a mineral corticoid hormone that regulates sodium and water in the body. The second is a glucocorticoid called *cortisol,* which increases blood glucose levels and helps regulate inflammation in the body. The third are the gonadotropin hormones: *testosterone, estrogen,* and *progesterone,* which are made in small amounts in both genders. These hormones will be covered in a later section.

The *medulla* secretes the adrenaline hormones *epinephrine* and *norepinephrine.* They are the hormones that respond to the sympathetic nervous system during times of stress. Often this is called the "fight or flight" response. In a life-threatening situation, we get a hormonal burst of energy. Fortunately, fight or flight is not normally a problem in our day-to-day society. Instead, we have traded acute life-threatening stress for chronic low grade, or at times chronic high-grade stress. Many of us are living with chronic stress and our bodies react like we are constantly being threatened. The problem is that we are not meant to constantly releasing adrenaline hormones and keeping our systems on high alert. Eventually these hormones become depleted. The first stage of adrenal hormone depletion is called *adrenal stress*. As the stress continues, *adrenal insufficiency* sets in and then finally *adrenal exhaustion*. Note that the term *adrenal fatigue* is no longer preferred.

Adrenal stress

The first stage of problems with adrenal hormones is called *adrenal stress*. This is what people mean when they say they feel "stressed." I call this the "tired but wired" phase. People feel pressure but have energy to push through the stress. They may feel tired but they do not sleep well (the classic pattern is waking in the middle of the night around 3:00 a.m. and not being able to get back to sleep; the stress causes an increase in the natural spike of hormones that wakes the body too much to fall back asleep). A lot of anxiety can exist in this phase. Many people fight through the pressure with caffeine and other stimulants, which ultimately increases the development of adrenal stress by further depleting stores of hormones.

Adrenal insufficiency

Adrenal insufficiency and adrenal exhaustion resulting from long-term emotional and physical stress are, unfortunately, very common today. Women preparing to get pregnant often have careers, husbands, family and social networks to maintain. Pregnancy, although a positive event in women's lives, is a major emotional and physical stress on the body. Addressing fatigue and exhaustion before pregnancy is important for a healthier pregnancy and baby.

Most women exhibiting fatigue and exhaustion symptoms are in fact suffering from adrenal insufficiency.

Although adrenal insufficiency is common, it is important to rule out much less common diseases that produce similar symptoms. Usually these other diseases are caused by a genetic absence of adrenal hormones, or autoimmune destruction as seen in Addison's disease.

Symptoms of adrenal stress

- Excessive fatigue or exhaustion
- Not feeling rested after sleeping
- Difficulty coping with stress

- Low endurance
- Difficulty recovering from exercise; feeling more tired with exercise
- Low immune function
- Poor digestion
- Multiple allergies and sensitivities to foods and chemicals in the environment
- Pre-Menstrual Syndrome (PMS) or increased menopausal symptoms
- Depression symptoms
- Difficulty concentrating
- Brain fog
- Low blood pressure
- Sensitivity to cold
- Slow recovery from illness or injury

Adrenal exhaustion

The next stage following adrenal insufficiency is *adrenal exhaustion or burnout* from chronic stress in our lives. Sometimes this is called *hypoadrenalism*, but this term is not always recognized by traditional physicians. The same symptoms of adrenal stress are present but they are more severe. People at this stage may be diagnosed with chronic fatigue, or fibromyalgia, and may live with severe fatigue, infections and pain. They often have digestive problems and issues with their thyroid and reproductive hormones.

Adrenal hormone concerns with pregnancy and infants

If a woman goes into pregnancy with, or during pregnancy has, adrenal stress (or adrenal insufficiency or exhaustion), it will affect her health and the health of her developing baby. Adrenal stress often leads to digestive problems with increased malabsorption of food and nutritional deficiencies. There is decreased immunity with a corresponding increased risk of infections. Increased allergies and sensitivities occur, which leads to increased inflammation and alteration of the immune system. Subsequently, the infant is born in a weakened state of health with an increased risk of infection, allergies, and inflammation, all which are seen more frequently in children with autism.

Lab evaluation

Adrenal hormone levels change throughout the day. Levels of cortisol tend to be higher in the morning and decrease throughout the day, which makes testing for them difficult.

Some physicians check cortisol levels via a blood draw. It is best to draw the blood in the morning. If it is low, especially in the morning when it should be at its high point, this is a good indication of adrenal fatigue. A morning blood level under 10 is significant even though a lab will label it as normal. There are more accurate methods for checking hormone levels. Saliva samples taken throughout the day track the normal pattern of cortisol. This is a common panel done by integrative practitioners and there are several labs that perform this test. Saliva samples are taken first thing in the morning then at lunch, dinner, and bedtime. A normal pattern is to have high levels in the morning and then decrease progressively until bedtime. We want to wake up in the morning and have energy and then by bedtime be relaxed enough to fall asleep.

Treatment

Adrenal stress in early stages can be treated easily. Later chronic stages often require the help of an integrative practitioner. As a first step, sources of stress should be reduced or eliminated as much as possible. Quitting a demanding job or leaving difficult relatives isn't usually an option, but simplifying life can be. Fewer commitments and more downtime is a great start. Exercise is a wonderful way to reduce stress. Research studies have determined that yoga and meditation reduce stress hormones and increase calming neurotransmitters in the brain such as GABA.[4]

Most women considering pregnancy would benefit from supplementation of vitamins and herbs that combat adrenal stress. The adrenal glands require a high amount of B and C vitamins, so adding these is an easy step before pregnancy. A multi-B vitamin complex containing on average 50 mg of each B vitamin a day is good, although some people will do better on 100 mg. A woman can usually take several grams of vitamin C per day as well.

Many single herbs or combination products are very supportive for the adrenals and work well with the vitamins. Herbs in these formulas are called *adaptogenic*, which means they bring the body to balance. Within the adaptogenic herbs, some are more energizing and some are more calming. Energizing herbs can be helpful for people in the more tired, dragging later stages of adrenal fatigue. Yet these same herbs can be anxiety provoking in those people in the "tired but wired" phase. Calming, balancing herbs are usually good for all people. Combination adrenal support formulas include multiple herbs that work well together. Adrenal glandulars are products that use adrenal glands from animals, and are found in supplements alone or with adrenal supporting herbs.

For women who show signs of adrenal stress, the additional physical requirements of supporting a healthy pregnancy and then nursing is often enough to tip them into adrenal insufficiency or exhaustion. Treatment before pregnancy is crucial. I recommend that women strengthen themselves before going into pregnancy, both for their health and the future health of their infant. Treatment for severe adrenal insufficiency/exhaustion can take months, so planning for this is important.

A treatment summary is listed below. Begin with the first item and proceed as needed, depending on level of adrenal fatigue.

Adrenal hormone treatment summary

1. Stress reduction
2. Exercise
3. Meditation
4. Additional sleep
5. Avoiding stimulants such as caffeine and certain herbs
6. Balancing blood sugar with low glycemic diet (the blood sugar roller coaster puts stress on adrenals and worsens issues)
7. Increased vitamin C
8. Increased vitamin B complex
9. Adrenal herbal support (individually or in combination) - examples: ginseng, ashwaganda, rhodiola, schisandra, Chinese herbs, and licorice
10. Acupuncture

11. Supplementing with adrenal glandulars: (from animals) usually with adaptogenic herbs (it is best to work with an integrative practitioner when using these products)

Thyroid Hormones

The thyroid produces hormones called *T3* and *T4*. They control other hormones and are our key regulators for metabolism. They inform our body how quickly to use energy. Thyroid hormones are important in children because they guide growth and development.

The thyroid hormones T3 and T4 are made in our bodies and require the mineral iodine and the amino acid tyrosine. If thyroid hormone levels are too low, someone is *hypothyroid*. When thyroid hormone levels are too high, the person is *hyperthyroid*. Hypothyroid disease is much more common and is becoming increasingly more common. Many toxins in our environment are hormone mimickers that impair thyroid function.

The release of hormones from the thyroid gland is controlled by two additional hormones. The *thyroid-stimulating hormone (TSH)* is produced by the anterior pituitary gland in the brain and directly controls the release of thyroid hormones. TSH itself is regulated by the *thyrotropin-releasing hormone (TRH)* that is produced in a structure in the brain called the *hypothalamus*.

Low thyroid (hypothyroid) symptoms

- Cold sensitivity (lower metabolic rate and lower body temperature)
- Fatigue or feeling worn down
- Depression
- Dry skin and eventually puffy swollen skin on face (myxedema)
- Weight gain
- Heavier menstrual periods in women
- Weakness
- Joint and/or muscle pain
- Constipation
- Brain fog

Elevated thyroid (hyperthyroid)

Elevated thyroid hormones cause the opposite symptoms from hypothyroid, and are less common. Metabolism is too high, which can result in weight loss and skipped or irregular heartbeats. One of the classic signs of hyperthyroid is protruding eyes. Sometimes people can develop hyperthyroid symptoms and then, as time goes by, deplete the hormones and become hypothyroid.

Thyroid hormone concerns with pregnancy and infants

It is well accepted that thyroid hormones are needed for cognitive development in infants during and after pregnancy. During pregnancy, especially early in pregnancy, the mother needs an adequate amount of thyroid hormone for proper nervous system development[6] and fetal growth.[7] Without this hormone, a child can suffer developmental delays in intellect, speech, and motor skills.[8,9] All of these delays are seen in children with autism. Low thyroid hormones in a mother can also lead to miscarriage and premature delivery.[10] It is also known that low thyroid levels can contribute to infertility.[11]

Low thyroid problems in a newborn, called *congenital hypothyroidism*, can lead to serious mental retardation, but fortunately we screen for this right after birth.[12] If a child has congenital hypothyroidism, they will require treatment with thyroid hormones for life.

In children with developmental or growth delays, I often screen for thyroid disorders. These children do not have the classic congenital hypothyroidism but have evidence of low thyroid function. Often these children also have decreased adrenal hormones. From the medical history, I often find their mother has diagnosed thyroid disease, symptoms of low thyroid or adrenal hormones, or a family history of thyroid problems. Treating these children with appropriate thyroid medication leads to improvements in development, growth, and energy. Ideally, women would be screened for thyroid problems before pregnancy, in order to prevent health problems in their children.

Thyroid hormone lab testing

It has been debated for decades whether all pregnant women should be screened for thyroid disorders. Research showing negative effects from missed thyroid disease favor universal screening.[13,14] Currently only high risk women are screened. High risk women are those with a personal history of thyroid disorder, family history of thyroid disorder, goiter (an enlarged thyroid gland), history of a blood test with positive thyroid antibodies, signs/symptoms of thyroid problems, type 1 diabetes, autoimmune disease, infertility, radiation to the head/neck, miscarriage or preterm delivery. The problem with this is that women with subclinical hypothyroid disease where no symptoms are seen but blood tests are positive still have an increased risk of miscarriage and negative effects on development.[15,16]

The initial screening for thyroid disorders checks TSH (thyroid stimulating hormone), which is the feedback hormone, not the direct thyroid hormone. The problem with this has to do with the unique thyroid hormone pathway for a fetus in the first trimester of pregnancy. During the first trimester, the fetus is unable to make its own thyroid hormones. The only thyroid hormone that can help the development of the infant's brain is the T4 hormone from the mother. Usually T4 is converted to T3, and it is T3 that has the direct effect on the organ. A normal T3 level in a mother will not prevent cognitive damage in a baby if her T4 hormone level is low. However, if T4 is low but T3 is normal, the TSH may also be normal, yet the cognitive development of the infant could still be impaired. The key point is that both free T4 and TSH need to be checked.

It is also important to check blood levels for *thyroid peroxidase antibody* (TPO-Ab) and a protein called *thyroglobulin-Ab* (Tg-Ab). These tests can provide early indication of autoimmune or other types of thyroid disease. Women can have positive autoimmune antibodies without thyroid disease, and be at increased risk of miscarriage.[17]

While the current debate is over whether to screen for thyroid disease when women are pregnant, I think this is the wrong debate. We need to screen women *before* pregnancy. Since an adequate amount of thyroid hormone is so important in the first trimester for an infant's cognitive development, screening at the end of the first trimester when a woman first knows she is pregnant is too late. Again, we need to go back before pregnancy and identify thyroid disease. This will decrease the potential fertility problems that some women might encounter, plus improve the woman's health before pregnancy. This will also prevent developmental delays from decreased thyroid hormones seen in children with autism. A simple blood test will help prevent serious health issues for a mother and her child.

During one of my prepregnancy workshops, two women had abnormal thyroid levels before pregnancy and were able to treat their hypothyroid disease before trying to conceive. This one test improved their fertility, pregnancy, and the health of their future child.

One of the problems with the testing is the interpretation of what is normal. A normal TSH in some labs is up to 4.0 or higher. Some endocrinologists and researchers consider any level of up to 2.0 to 3.5 or higher as abnormal, and a marker of hypothyroid. For women during pregnancy, it is recommended to keep the TSH at a lower level, below 2.5.[18,19] A woman may have a TSH of 3.7 and be considered normal by some labs, but her low thyroid hormone status may have a negative impact on her child. It is very important to know the actual level and for the mother to discuss it with a knowledgeable practitioner.

Another way to gather information on thyroid hormone status is to go back to our original method of testing basal body temperatures. This was done routinely before blood testing was available. A person's basal body temperature will be low if their thyroid hormones are low. Before getting out of bed in the morning, a person places a thermometer under their arm for 10 minutes and records the result. The thermometer should be similar to the traditional mercury thermometers where small increments can be read. This should be done for 5 days in a row. A normal body temperature is 97.8 to 98.2. Consistently low temperatures are indicative of hypothyroid disease.

Another critical component of thyroid function is having adequate amounts of the mineral iodine. Iodine was traditionally put in salt in order to prevent thyroid problems. Some of the sea salts that people use today do not have enough iodine, although prenatal vitamins have the additional amounts needed in pregnancy.

<u>Summary of laboratory testing for thyroid disorders</u>

- TSH (thyroid stimulating hormone)
- Free T4 hormone level
- TPO-Ab (thyroid peroxidase antibody) and Tg-Ab (thyroglobulin-Ab)
- Basal body temperature

Treatment for abnormal thyroid hormones

If thyroid hormones are low, usually the adrenal hormones are weak. It is important to begin treatment of low adrenal hormones first, otherwise a person can have a negative reaction to thyroid treatment. I have seen proper thyroid treatment stopped because of a negative reaction to a thyroid medication.

When treating the thyroid, it is important to have a good source of iodine (150 mcg a day) and selenium (50 mcg a day). Both of these minerals are crucial for the body's production of thyroid hormones. Adequate protein is also important.

If a woman has low thyroid before pregnancy, this needs to be treated. The safest most studied treatment is the prescription levothyroxine (common name *Synthroid*™).[20] While integrative practitioners frequently use a prescription containing both T3 and T4 in a glandular form, I not aware of any safety research for its use during pregnancy. Since the T4 hormone is also needed for the infant's brain development, at this point in time I consider levothyroxine the best choice during pregnancy.

Thyroid hormones are easily disrupted by toxins including heavy metals, (such as mercury), plastics, and paraben preservatives in cosmetics. Removing any potential hormone disruptors from a person's environment is another key step toward thyroid health. The remaining steps, which will be discussed in subsequent chapters, are strengthening the detoxification system and then detoxifying.

Steroid Hormones: Estrogen and Progesterone

The steroid hormones estrogen and progesterone are obviously crucial for a woman to become pregnant and then maintain the pregnancy. As stress increases, there is an order of how the hormones in the body are affected. First the adrenal hormones become depleted, then the thyroid hormones, and then eventually the steroid hormones. If a woman is experiencing infertility, the steroid hormones often will be evaluated. If they are elevated the next step is to test the adrenal and thyroid hormones.

Unfortunately, infertility issues are increasing in our country, in part because women are having babies at later ages. There are other factors as well. Some medical researchers are examining the large amounts of environmental toxins women are exposed to called *xenoestrogens* or estrogen mimickers. For some women these cause an imbalance between estrogen and progesterone leading to menstrual and fertility issues. These estrogen mimickers also affect men and reduce their fertility.

If effects from toxins are a problem, the answer is to clean up a person's environment and help their body detoxify (discussed in later chapters). If infertility is a problem, a woman should work with a qualified health care practitioner to address toxicity and hormone balance including adrenal, thyroid, and estrogen and progesterone levels. Acupuncture and Chinese herbs from a qualified practitioner can help.

Summary

Fertility and maintaining pregnancy rely on a balance of estrogen and progesterone. It is important to realize that the adrenal and thyroid hormones also play a role in this process and are intertwined with healthy estrogen and progesterone levels.

Today, with stress and toxic chemicals, it is easy for hormones to get disrupted. It is important to address hormone issues before pregnancy in order to have the best chance for a full term pregnancy and a healthy child.

CHAPTER 9 REFERENCES

1. Weinstock M. The potential influence of maternal stress hormones on development and mental health of the offspring. *Brain, Behavior, and Immunity.* 2005;19(4):296-308. DH479.

2. Ibid.

3. Kinney DK, Munir KM, Crowley DJ, Miller AM. Prenatal stress and risk for autism. *Neurosci Biobehav Rev.* 2008 Oct;32(8):1519-32. DH396.

4. Ibid.

5. Beddoe AE, Lee KA. Mind-body interventions during pregnancy. *J Obstet Gynecol Neonatal Nurs.* 2008 Mar-Apr;37(2):165-75. DH399.

6. Henrichs J, Bongers-Schokking JJ, Schenk JJ, Ghassabian A, Schmidt HG, Visser TJ, Hooijkaas H, de Muinck Keizer-Schrama SM, Hofman A, Jaddoe VV, Visser W, Steegers EA, Verhulst FC, de Rijke YB, Tiemeier H. Maternal thyroid function during early pregnancy and cognitive functioning in early childhood: the generation R study. *J Clin Endocrinol Metab.* 2010 Sep;95(9):4227-34. DH410.

7. Männistö T, Vääräsmäki M, Pouta A, Hartikainen AL, Ruokonen A, Surcel HM, Bloigu A, Järvelin MR, Suvanto-Luukkonen E. Perinatal outcome of children born to mothers with thyroid dysfunction or antibodies: a prospective population-based cohort study. *J Clin Endocrinol Metab.* 2009 Mar;94(3):772-9. DH413.

8. Henrichs 2010.

9. Pop VJ, Kuijpens JL, van Baar AL, Verkerk G, van Son MM, de Vijlder JJ, Vulsma T, Wiersinga WM, Drexhage HA, Vader HL. Low maternal free thyroxine concentrations during early pregnancy are associated with impaired psychomotor development in infancy. *Clin Endocrinol (Oxf).* 1999 Feb;50(2):149-55. DH418.

10. Su PY, Huang K, Hao JH, Xu YQ, Yan SQ, Li T, Xu YH, Tao FB. Maternal thyroid function in the first twenty weeks of pregnancy and subsequent fetal and infant development: a prospective population-based cohort study in China. *J Clin Endocrinol Metab.* 2011 Oct;96(10):3234-41. DH412.

11. Rijal B, Shrestha R, Jha B. Association of thyroid dysfunction among infertile women visiting infertility center of Om Hospital, Kathmandu, Nepal. *Nepal Med Coll J.* 2011 Dec;13(4):247-9. DH481.

12. Abduljabbar MA, Afifi AM. Congenital hypothyroidism. *J Pediatr Endocrinol Metab.* 2012;25(1-2):13-29. DH482.

13. Budenhofer BK, Ditsch N, Jeschke U, Gärtner R, Toth B. Thyroid (dys-) function in normal and disturbed pregnancy. *Arch Gynecol Obstet.* 2013 Jan;287(1):1-7.

14. Lepoutre T, Debiève F, Gruson D, Daumerie C. Reduction of miscarriages through universal screening and treatment of thyroid autoimmune diseases. *Gynecol Obstet Invest.* 2012;74(4):265-73.

15. Ibid.

16. Stagnaro-Green A, Pearce E. Thyroid disorders in pregnancy. *Nat Rev Endocrinol.* 2012 Nov;8(11):650-8. DH575.

17. Lepoutre 2012.

18. Budenhofer 2013.

19. Garber JR, Cobin RH, Gharib H, Hennessey JV, Klein I, Mechanick JI, Pessah-Pollack R, Singer PA, Woeber KA; American Association of Clinical Endocrinologists and American Thyroid Association Taskforce on Hypothyroidism in Adults. Clinical practice guidelines for hypothyroidism in adults: cosponsored by the American Association of Clinical Endocrinologists and the American Thyroid Association. *Endocr Pract.* 2012 Nov-Dec;18(6):988-1028. DH576.

20. Ibid.

10

Environmental Toxins

After covering nutrition, digestion, and metabolism, it is now time to turn to the external environment. This is the third part of the Triangle of Prevention and it consists of two important components: (1) learning what toxins exist in our environment that can potentially harm a developing baby and how to best avoid them, and (2) strengthening the body and detoxifying safely. Since it is only safe to detoxify before pregnancy, detoxification is a crucial component of the preconception period.

The EPA estimates there are over 87,000 chemicals used commercially in the U.S. How many of these chemicals have been tested for their effects on pregnant women and children? How many of these chemicals have been tested together or tested for long-term effects? Unfortunately, few of them have. The studies that have been done were completed after the chemicals were put on the market and focus on non-pregnant adults. Their effects on our most vulnerable populations of pregnant women and children have not been studied adequately.

Our modern environment causes exposure to multiple chemicals every day—many of which have toxins harmful to human health. Avoiding all toxins in our environment is impossible in today's world. Women carry these toxins and then pass them to their babies even before birth or later while nursing. Research from the Environmental Working Group showed an average of 200 toxins measured in cord blood from newborn infants.[1] These toxins include toxins that are known to cause cancer, harm the nervous system, and cause abnormal development. They even found evidence of toxins such as *dichlorodiphenyltrichloroethane (DDT)* that have been banned in the U.S. for decades.[2]

While we cannot fully separate ourselves from all of the chemicals around us, we can control some of the exposure. We need to identify which toxins are the worst offenders and avoid them as much as possible. For existing exposures, we need to help strengthen the body and promote its natural ability to detoxify. Finally, women planning to get pregnant should be educated in methods to help remove some of the toxins before attempting to get pregnant since it is not safe to detoxify once pregnant or when nursing.

Exposure

Chemical exposure happens when toxins enter the body. For example, breathing contaminated air will bring pollutants into the lungs. Food and water can be unsuspected toxin sources; aluminum in baking soda, arsenic in water, and mercury in high fructose corn syrup[3] are all sources many people would not even consider. Chemicals can even be absorbed through the skin.

Toxin exposure can be sudden (a splash of gasoline on the hand) or a low dose over an extended time (mercury in the air we breathe from a coal-fired power plant). Quantifying exposure is important because it is often the cumulative amount of chemicals that determines the impact. This is the concept of *toxic burden*. The higher the amount of toxins a person retains, the higher that person's toxic burden. Since toxins can be passed through the placenta and breast milk, an infant's toxic burden begins even before birth. Therefore, a child's toxic burden begins with the toxins of the mother.

The effects from toxins vary because some chemicals are more harmful than others. For example, a small amount of a dangerous metal such as mercury is more harmful than a larger amount of a metal such as tin. This is the idea behind the old adage that *the dose makes the poison.* Even substances that are usually good for us such as water can be toxic if the dose is too high.

Toxins in combination can be more harmful than toxins individually. This is *potentiation,* where the toxicity of one chemical is increased by another chemical. For example, one chemical destroys the liver enzyme that is needed for detoxifying another chemical. The chemicals don't even have to be present at the same time. Another concern is that when some chemicals combine in water or other areas of the environment they can form new harmful chemicals. An example of this was found at the Rocky Mountain Arsenal in Colorado. A new chemical was discovered in the ground water that was never used at the arsenal.[4]

Toxins also enter the foods we eat. They concentrate as they pass up the food chain with humans being on the top, for example when pesticides sprayed on lakes enter fish that are later consumed by humans.

How Toxins Cause Harm

Toxins harm the body in multiple ways. Understanding the basic biochemistry of how this happens is helpful in understanding how harmful a chemical can be.

The first way that toxins may cause harm is damage to the nervous system. These toxins are called *neurotoxins.* For a developing nervous system in utero, and then for a young child, these chemicals are extremely dangerous. Below is a list of *known* toxins that have been shown to harm the nervous system and lead to developmental delays.

Chemicals associated with neurodevelopmental disabilities (neurotoxic chemicals)

- Lead
- Mercury
- Polychlorinated biphenyl (PCBs)
- Arsenic
- Manganese
- Organophosphate pesticides
- Dichlorodiphenyltrichloroethane (DDT)
- Ethanol (alcohol)

The above list includes only *known* neurotoxins. This list doesn't take into account the many chemicals that are *suspected* neurotoxins. Thousands of other chemicals may be neurotoxic, but we do not know because of inadequate testing.

Chemicals can also have negative hormone health effects on both the mother and baby. They can act like estrogen and have hormone -promoting action, such as bisphenol A (BPA). These are called *xenoestrogens*. They can also block hormone function (e.g. hypothyroid). We know little about the effects of these chemicals on pregnancy hormonal regulation or the impact on the fetus.

We know that autism is much more common in boys. How are these chemicals with hormonal effects playing a role in our gender discrepancy in this disease? We urgently need to find out.

Toxic chemicals can also dangerously affect our genetic material (DNA) by causing direct damage, or by changing how the DNA is controlled. Chemicals that cause a direct effect on DNA can lead to cancer and are called *carcinogenic* chemicals. Chemicals that lead to birth defects by changing the DNA in a fetus are called *mutagenic* chemicals. Chemicals can be both carcinogenic and mutagenic depending on the time of exposure. Changes to the control of DNA expression are called *epigenetic* effects. Numerous chemicals appear to have epigenetic effects.

Since chemicals are foreign substances in the body, they can trigger allergic reactions by disrupting the immune system. If a person breathes a chemical, it can trigger asthma or a chronic cough. A chemical put on the skin can cause a skin rash. Ingested chemicals can cause a wide variety of allergic reactions, including digestive problems, as well as difficulty in breathing and skin rashes (even though the chemicals did not have direct contact with the lungs or the skin). Sometimes chemicals can cause reactions that trigger the immune system in a different way. They can cause the body to have an immune reaction against itself (an autoimmune reaction). Children with autism exhibit many similar problems with their immune system including antibodies against their own tissues.[5] We need to understand better how the toxins are involved with this process.

Unique Susceptibility

One of the most concerning effects of toxins is their unique effect on children. Children are not just small adults. They are immature beings in the process of growing and developing. We all know babies do not come out walking and talking, yet many people expect their immature bodies to process chemicals in the same way as adults do. Since they are smaller in weight, one dose of a toxin that is not dangerous in an adult could be very harmful for a baby who is $1/10^{th}$ the size, or on a fetus weighing just a few ounces.

According to the National Institute of Environmental Health Sciences (NIEHS), chemicals and pollutants that "may have minimal effects on adults may impact the developing fetus and have long-lasting effects on a child's health even into adulthood." [6] This is called the *fetal basis of adult disease.*

The timing and duration of toxin exposure during fetal or infant development largely determines its health effect, called the toxicant's *windows of vulnerability.* Fetal organs develop at different rates and are particularly susceptible to toxins at certain critical times.[7] The research article *Children's Susceptibility to Toxicants* by Faustman EM, et. al.[8] gives excellent examples of how toxins harm normal cellular development/replication during pregnancy and how (from rodent studies) varying toxin exposure by just a few days during pregnancy can determine whether there will be birth defects.

Without adequate research on the vulnerability of mother, fetus, and infant to toxic substances, the EPA currently uses a default multiplier of 10 for exposure limits for pregnant women, when in fact risks may be several orders of magnitude greater during certain periods of fetal/infant development.[9] As an example, a pregnant woman getting an abdominal x-ray during week four of pregnancy may endanger her fetus, although the radiation exposure would be well within normal toxin exposure limits to adults.

When a child is exposed to chemicals, the chemicals come into direct contact with a nervous system that is in the process of developing and forming new nerve connections. The chemicals are neurotoxic and harm normal development.

All people have a protective mechanism in their nervous system called the *blood brain barrier* that tries to block dangerous chemicals from entering the brain. It is unclear from research whether infants are born with a fully intact blood brain barrier or whether it takes months to years to develop.

The digestive system also has protective mechanisms to prevent ingested toxins from entering the rest of the body. The intestine has a barrier lining to prevent toxins from passing into the body. When the lining is not intact, it is called *leaky gut* or *intestinal hyperpermeabilty*. Infants are not born with a fully developed digestive system and so therefore are more at risk from toxins in food. After birth, infections can also break down the intestinal lining leading to a leaky gut. Even medicines such as ibuprofen or steroids can damage the intestinal lining.

There are gender differences in toxin susceptibility. Since each gender has different amounts of the reproductive hormones (estrogen, progesterone, and testosterone) they react differently to chemicals. It is thought that estrogen is protective for some substances, since autism is much less prevalent in girls. One theory is that estrogen acts protectively against some of the environmental toxin exposures.

Detoxification

The body is designed with several detoxification systems to detect and rid itself of chemicals. The primary systems are the digestive system, (which includes the liver and the intestines) and the renal system (the kidneys).

The liver is the body's primary detoxification organ. Toxins in the blood stream pass through the liver and are changed by chemical detoxification reactions into substances that are less harmful and can be eliminated from the body. These detoxification reactions can be overwhelmed if there are too many toxins passing through the liver. There are also genetic differences of how many toxins a person can process, called *genetic polymorphisms*. These can be tested through specific detoxification test panels.

The kidneys, lungs, and skin are also important organs of toxin elimination. The kidneys need to reabsorb some nutrients and eliminate others to keep steady amounts of nutrients in the blood. They eliminate toxins through the urinary tract. Again, an infant is not born with a renal or kidney system that is fully developed and able to handle excessive toxins.

The lungs exhale carbon dioxide (CO2) and other toxins and the skin sweats-out toxins. If the liver and digestive system are not fully functional or have reached their detoxifying capacity, many substances will be excreted through the skin. This is the reason skin rashes are more common in childhood.

If the body isn't able to eliminate the toxins, it stores them to get them out of the blood stream and lessen the acute harm. Some toxins, such as lead, are stored in bone tissue. Other toxins, such as mercury, are stored in the brain, heart, and kidneys. Many pesticides and other similar chemicals are stored in fat tissues because they are fat-soluble compounds. Once the chemicals are stored, they can still harm body tissues and tend to cause long term or chronic problems. They are also more difficult to remove from the body.

The EPA, Contaminants, and Children

In 1998, the Endocrine Disruptor Screening and Testing Advisory Committee made recommendations to the EPA that the 87,000 chemicals used be "considered for endocrine disruptor screening and testing."[10] Two decades later the EPA is only now developing a "strategy" for determining the health impacts of these tens of thousands of chemicals.[11]

To advise policymakers and protect human health, the EPA released in January 2013 the third edition of the report *"America's Children and the Environment."* Interestingly, the 2011 draft version of this report met with strong resistance from the chemical industry.[12]

The report states the following in the Neurodevelopmental Disorders section:

> "A child's brain and nervous system are vulnerable to adverse impacts from pollutants because they go through a long developmental process beginning shortly after conception and continuing through adolescence. This complex developmental process requires the precise coordination of cell growth and movement, and may be disrupted be even short-term exposures to environmental contaminants if they occur at critical stages of development. This disruption can lead to neurodevelopmental deficits..."

The report discusses the causes of ADHD:

> *"While uncertainties remain, findings to date indicate that ADHD is caused by combinations of genetic and environmental factors. Much of the research on environmental factors has focused on the fetal environment. ... The potential role of environmental contaminants in contributing to ADHD, either alone or in conjunction with certain genetic susceptibilities or other environmental factors, is becoming better understood as a growing number of studies look explicitly at the relationship between ADHD and exposures to environmental contaminants."*

It states the following for Autism Spectrum Disorders:

> *"To date, no single risk factor sufficient to cause ASD has been identified; rather each case is likely to be caused by the combination of multiple risk factors. Several ASD research findings and hypotheses may imply an important role for environmental contaminants. First, there has been a sharp upward trend in prevalence that cannot be fully explained by younger ages at diagnosis, migration patterns, changes in diagnostic criteria, inclusion of milder cases or increased parental age. Also, the neurological signaling systems that are impaired in children with ASDs can be affected by certain environmental chemicals.*
>
> *Furthermore, many of the identified genetic risk factors for autism are de novo mutations, meaning that the genetic defect is not present in either of the parents' genes, yet can be found in the genes of the child when a new genetic mutation forms in a parent's germ cells (egg or sperm), potentially from exposure to contaminants. These de novo mutations in autistic children have been found in the genes that are involved in the structure or function of nervous system synapses.*
>
> *Many studies have linked increasing paternal and maternal age with increased risk of ASDs. The role of parental age in increased autism risk may be explained by evidence that shows advanced parental age to contribute significantly to the frequency of de novo mutations in a parent's germ cells. Advanced parental age signifies a longer period of time when environmental exposures may act on germ cells and cause DNA damage and de novo mutations."*

"Proximity to industrial and power plant sources of environmental mercury has been linked to increased autism prevalence in a study conducted in Texas."

The Polluting "P's"

Understanding how toxins affect women and children is the first step in helping improve the health of children. Since discussing each one of the 87,000 chemicals is overwhelming for women contemplating pregnancy, the next step is to learn about the worst offenders. I assign the most harmful chemicals into a group called the *Polluting P's*. The Polluting P's contain many chemicals in our daily environment along with many in beauty products that contact our skin.

Pesticides

The Polluting P's begin with pesticides. We often come into contact with them from our food, although we have to remember that they are also sprayed on our yards and gardens. Pesticides were discussed in Chapter 5 under *Foods to Avoid.*

Petrochemicals

Petrochemicals are products made from petroleum. These chemicals are ever-present in our environment, whether from preservatives in cosmetics, to packaging of foods, and even to some of the clothing we wear. Petrochemicals have been widely used for the past 50 years and most women today have been exposed to them their entire lives. We do not fully know the long-term impact of many of these substances. What we do know is that many of them have hormonal effects causing problems with estrogen and thyroid hormones. Others are toxic to the development of the nervous system. We need to determine if there is a connection between the large increase in exposure to these substances and the increasing problems with fertility and the declining health of our children. I strongly suspect there is.

Plastics

Plastics are ubiquitous in our environment and are a type of petrochemical. Exposure can be from plastic fumes, plastic in clothing (polyester), or from ingestion of food wrapped in plastic packaging or heated in plastic containers. Plastic can even contaminate the water we drink from plastic water bottles.

There are many ways in which plastics can cause harm. They can be carcinogenic or cause hypersensitivity reactions. A primary concern for women and children is plastic's ability to act as an endocrine disruptor.

There are two main types of plastics. They have different chemical structures and cause different health effects.

Thermoplastics

Thermoplastics become soft when heated and then harden when cooled. These are plastics that are flexible but dangerous to our health because they emit vapors (called *off-gassing*) that we inhale. One of the most dangerous plastics in this category is vinyl chloride or polyvinyl chloride (PVC). Examples of PVCs include shower curtains, plastic toys such as beach balls, containers for cosmetics, and vinyl flooring. A recent study examining causes of autism found increased risks of autism in children with exposure to vinyl floors.[13] This was an unexpected finding since the study was not specifically looking at PVCs. Women preparing for pregnancy should avoid vinyl floors. Baby toys such as pacifiers are still being made from PVCs. Common sense should dictate that a young vulnerable infant should not chew on plastic. Fortunately, plastics are being used less in some young children's toys.

Thermoplastics include acrylic plastics made from acrylonitrile (a suspected carcinogen), polyethylene, and the fluorocarbon plastic called *polytetrafluoroethylene* known as Teflon on non-stick pans. Teflon emits toxic vapors when heated and since it is common to heat a pan when cooking this is a serious safety issue. In 2003, the Environmental Working Group petitioned the U.S. Consumer Product Safety Commission to attach warning labels to cookware with non-stick coatings due to documented cases of bird deaths and concern for human health.[14] Safer pans are available made from ceramic or other coatings.

One of the final types of thermoplastics is widely known as Styrofoam. Styrofoam is made from polystyrene or a combination called *ABS (acrylonitrile/butadiene/styrene)*. It mimics estrogen, disrupts thyroid hormone function, and is neurotoxic. Think of all the coffee cups and carryout containers that people are exposed to over a lifetime made out of Styrofoam.

We even have clothes made out of plastic. Polyester is plastic clothing. Many of the light fabrics we have are made with plastic chemicals.

Thermosets

The second type of plastic covered in this section is called thermosets. These chemicals begin as soft plastics but when heated, their shape is set. They are safer in general than thermoplastics because they do not off-gas. There are two dangerous exceptions in this category: (1) urea-formaldehyde used in building materials such as particleboard and plywood which outgasses and is a human carcinogen,[15] and (2) polyurethane foam used in furniture and pillows which can cause lung problems. Shouldn't people know if a pillow where their head is resting every night could cause them lung problems in the future?

Plastics Recommendations

It should be obvious from the above that we are exposed to multiple types of plastics on a daily basis. Since some plastics are safer than others, we can rely on the recycling number on the bottom of containers to let us know which ones are safer—see Table 10.1. The safest plastic containers are numbers 2, 4, and 5. Yet, are these plastics really safe? Even though some types of plastics are considered safer, is that because we do not yet know the harm they actually cause? Since many of these substances are new to our environment in the last few decades and testing is limited, it may be too early to know for sure.

For a woman preparing for pregnancy, avoidance of plastics with the numbers 3, 6, and 7 is a good place to begin. The next step is getting rid of plastic water bottles: there are some better options such as glass and steel. This also preserves our environment from mountains of waste. If a plastic water bottle is needed, a woman should choose one that is BPA-free (see below for an explanation of BPAs).

Preventing plastics from coming in contact with food is a good practice. This includes not using takeout Styrofoam and leftover plastic storage containers. Women should not heat or microwave anything in plastic to avoid leaching toxins into food. Glass storage containers are a great investment. As a final precaution, Teflon-coated pans should be avoided.

Table 10.1 - Summary of Plastics

Plastic number	Safety	Material	Where found	Recycle?
#1	Adequate, but there is a concern with bacterial growth upon reuse	PETE or polyethylene terephthalate	Disposable soda and water bottles	Yes
#2	Safer	HDPE or high density polyethylene	Milk and juice containers, detergent bottles, butter tubs	Yes
#3	Avoid	PVC or polyvinyl chloride often with phthalates	Food wrap and plumbing pipes	No
#4	Safer	LDPE or low density polyethylene	Grocery bags, bread bags, squeezable bottles	No
#5	Safer	Polypropylene	Yogurt cups, medicine bottles, ketchup and syrup bottles, straws	No. May in the future
#6	Avoid	Styrofoam or polystyrene	Disposable containers and cups	No
#7	Caution	All other plastics: polycarbonate BPA (avoid)	Computer cases, parts of iPods, baby bottles, food storage containers, etc.	No

Bisphenol A (BPA)

Even though BPA is a type of plastic, it deserves special attention because of the profound negative impact it can have on pregnant women and children. BPA was originally developed as an estrogen hormone receptor medicine. Now it is a common ingredient in baby bottles! How it traveled from a hormone medicine to a common ingredient in baby bottles should be concerning. The European Union banned BPA in baby bottles in 2011.[16]

In 2012, the U.S. Food and Drug Administration prohibited the use of BPA in baby bottles. The only way to be certain that the bottle is safe is if the label states that it is "BPA-free." Other sources of BPA include a wide array of uses from dental sealants, flame-retardants, lining of canned foods, and paper receipts from everyday purchases. A total of 93% of the U.S. population have been exposed to BPA based on urine samples done from the National Health and Nutrition Examination Survey.[17] Unfortunately exposures appear to be even higher in women compared to men, and children compared to adults.[18]

In addition to hormone concerns, BPA has effects on neurodevelopment. It has been shown in studies to interfere with both estrogen and thyroid hormones with particular concern to pregnant women, fetuses, and small children.[19] These hormones adversely affect sperm and may increase the risk of testicular cancer.[20] For women, research has shown associations with a range of issues including recurrent miscarriages and breast cancer.[21]

For preventing autism and ADHD, avoidance of BPA appears to be crucial. Research has shown negative emotional and cognitive effects of BPA in animals and humans. Animal studies have shown problems in nervous system tissue important in memory, learning, and emotions with doses considered safe in humans.[22] Research is now focusing more on neurodevelopmental effects on children. A study published in 2012 showed a correlation between a child's exposure to BPA in utero and emotional and behavior issues between the ages of 3-5 years.[23] A higher exposure to BPA in utero was associated with more problems on emotionally reactive and aggressive behavior syndromes. Of importance is that boys had a more significant negative impact from the BPA than girls.

With its negative effects on both hormones and neurodevelopment, BPA is doubly dangerous. The bottom line is that all women considering pregnancy should entirely avoid this substance.

Solvents

Solvents are another group of chemicals produced from petroleum. This includes xylene, toluene, benzene, and styrene. Solvents give off fumes, which is one of the primary ways people are exposed. We know that styrene is the solvent used to make the plastic Styrofoam. The solvent xylene is one of the most common petrochemicals and is a primary pollutant in smog. Toluene is another common solvent used as an additive in gasoline. It is also present in nail polish.

All of these solvents are neurotoxins and therefore dangerous to a developing child. In addition, concern is raised about their effects on endocrine hormones and their ability to promote cancer. There are urine tests that look at a person's exposure to these solvents in addition to the chemicals phthalates and parabens present in cosmetics. This test needs to be interpreted by a knowledgeable practitioner because test results showing low levels may mean that there is a problem getting rid of the chemicals – not actual low levels of exposure.

Polychlorinated Biphenyls (PCBs)

PCBs are a type of organochlorine compound similar to dioxin and other pesticides. Even though these chemicals were banned in the 1970s, they are still found in people tested for pollutants today. They are a type of persistent organic pollutant since they are difficult to remove fully from the environment. Currently, they still pollute some of our water and therefore our fish. In humans, PCBs deposit in fat tissue, which is a concern, since women mobilize fat to produce breast milk for their infant. In a similar manner to pesticides, they disrupt hormone function and are toxic to the nervous system.

Perchlorates (e.g. Perchloroethylene)

These chemicals are used in dry cleaning and spot removers. They are solvents and cause fumes that are carcinogenic and often cause sleepiness, dizziness, light-headedness, and disorientation. Extremely high doses can be fatal. Luckily there are healthier choices with dry cleaners using CO_2 or silicone-based techniques.

Cleaning Products

Many toxic chemicals exist in our everyday cleaning products. If the product has a hazard symbol on the bottle, avoid it. Any cleaner that has potent fumes coming from the bottle should be avoided. There are many safer products that actually smell good and are made from natural essential oils. Even basic kitchen ingredients such as vinegar and lemon are safe and effective cleaners.

Coal Tar

Neither the word "coal" nor "tar" beckons the consumer. However, coal tar is an ingredient in many consumer products, such as shampoos. As you would guess, coal tar is derived from processing of coal. The primary concern is that this substance contains over 10,000 different chemicals, with 50% of them unidentified.[24] Chemicals verified in coal tar include a class of chemicals called *polycyclic aromatic hydrocarbons* that have been shown to cause cancer.[25] Other chemicals include solvents such as benzene and xylene, toxins such as naphthalene (an ingredient in moth balls), phenol, and creosol. Many of them have toxicity concerns including cancer, allergies, and inhibition of the immune system. Other coal tar chemicals are linked to skin irritation and breathing problems.

Coal tar is sometimes used in asphalt paving. During the hot paving process, dangerous polycyclic aromatic hydrocarbons are released into the air that people breathe. Several cities and states have banned its use in asphalt but its use in other products exists. The construction industry uses multiple products that contain coal tar including wall insulation, roofs, boilers, and fabric dyes.

Unseen Hazards: Electromagnetic Fields (EMFs)

There has been a large increase in our exposure to electromagnetic fields with the use of wireless technology, cell phones, microwaves, and electricity used in the home. Most people spend the majority of the day closely exposed to EMFs from computer and cell phone use.

Humans have their own electromagnetic energy in the body: for example, we measure the heart's electrical energy by EKGs (electrocardiogram) and the brain's electrical waves from an EEG (electroencephalogram).

Research is only beginning on the health effects of EMFs. There are many issues to be examined. What are the effects on the brain of having a cell phone pressed against it many times a day for years on end? Children absorb more radiation and now they are using these devices from a young age. This is frightening.

It appears that EMFs decrease the production of melatonin.[26] Melatonin is the chemical in the body that regulates sleep rhythms and is an important precursor for the calming neurotransmitter, serotonin. Fertility may also be negatively impacted. Men who carry cell phones in their pockets appear to have decreased sperm viability.[27] Obviously for any couple trying to get pregnant, this is an important consideration. It may affect the integrity of our DNA.[28] Children with higher amounts of cell phone exposure beginning in utero appear to have an increase in emotional and behavioral issues.[29] Finally, concern has been raised about the increased risk of brain tumors from having cell phones pressed to the head.[30]

There are additional sources of EMF health concerns on the web. Several manufacturers sell devices to shield us from EMFs. We definitely need to learn more about this important topic.

Pregnant women have traditionally been told to avoid x-rays during pregnancy. When I was pregnant and doing my hospital medical training, I remember running away from the portable X-ray machine. Now there is nowhere to run.

Basic safety from EMFs

- Use a speakerphone or headset with cell phones
- Avoid Bluetooth headsets (they concentrate EMFs)
- Keep cell phones off the body
- Avoid cell phone use in cars, trains, and elevators (they concentrate EMFs)
- In the home, use hand-held landline phones
- Avoid wireless router or unplug at night
- Decrease exposure by removing electrical appliances in the bedroom. Don't sleep next to a cell phone, iPad, or electric alarm clock.
- Keep up with latest research

Air Pollution

Another unseen hazard is the air we breathe both inside our home, and outside in what we consider "fresh air." It appears that living near highways and industrial areas is associated with increased health risks. Researchers compared pregnant women's home addresses to the EPA's air quality monitoring location data. Traffic-related air pollution contains nitrogen dioxide and particle pollution called $PM_{2.5}$ and PM_{10}. In 2013, the researchers published a study that found that pregnant women exposed to traffic-related air pollution had increased incidence of autism[31] (yet another risk factor).

Even after children are born, the quality of the air can have negative effects on their neurodevelopment. A study showed that autism rates may be higher in areas with greater pollution (e.g. near EPA superfund sites).[32]

Indoor air can also contain many toxins from materials and chemicals used in the home. These pollutants can also harm children's health.[33]

Summary

Our world is full of chemicals with new ones being released continually. The goal of these chemicals is to advance our standard of living, but these modern conveniences come at a price. Unfortunately, the most vulnerable in our population, pregnant women and children, pay that price. Any woman considering pregnancy must take the precautionary route: not only do they need to avoid the many known harmful toxins, they need to avoid substances that *may* be harmful to their health and the health of their future child.

CHAPTER 10 REFERENCES

1. Environmental Working Group. Body Burden-The pollution in newborns: A benchmark investigation of industrial chemicals, pollutants, and pesticides in umbilical cord blood. *Environmental Working Group*. July 14, 2005. DH289.

2. Ibid.

3. Dufault R, LeBlanc B, Schnoll R, Cornett C, Schweitzer L, Wallinga D, Hightower J, Patrick L, Lukiw WJ. Mercury from chlor-alkali plants: measured concentrations in food product sugar. *Environ Health*. 2009 Jan 26;8:2. DH577.

4. Walton, G. Public Health Aspects of the Contamination of Ground Water in South Platte River Basin in Vicinity of Henderson, Colorado. U.S. Public Health Service. Nov 2, 1959. DH578.

5. Goines P, Van de Water J. The immune system's role in the biology of autism, *Curr Opin Neurol*. 2010 Apr;23(2):111-117. DH183.

6. U.S. Environmental Protection Agency. Universe of Chemicals and General Validation Principles. Office of Chemical Safety & Pollution Prevention, EPA publication. *EPA Endocrine Disruptor Screening Program*. 2012 Nov. DH484.

7. Mendola P, Selevan SG, Gutter S, Rice D. Environmental factors associated with a spectrum of neurodevelopmental deficits. *Ment Retard Dev Diabil Res Rev*. 2002;8(3):188-197. DH300.

8. Faustman EM, Silbernagel SM, Fenske RA, Burbacher TM, Ponce RA. 2000. Mechanisms underlying children's susceptibility to environmental toxicants. *Env Health Persp*. 2000. 108: Suppl 1:13 21. DH487.

9. Ibid.

10. EPA 2012.

11. EPA 2012.

12. Kaplan S. White House stalls critical EPA report highlighting chemicals dangers to children. *Amer Uni Investigative Reporting Workshop Investigation*. 2012 Dec 21. DH483.

13. Larsson M, Weiss B, Janson S, Sundell J, Bornehag CG. Associations between indoor environmental factors and parental-reported autistic spectrum disorders in children 6-8 years of age. *Neuro Tox*. Sep 2009;30(5)822-831. DH185.

14. Environmental Working Group. Petition to the U.S. Consumer Product Safety Commission to require warning labels on cookware and heated appliances bearing non-stick coatings. 2003 May 15. DH498.

15. Harris JC, Rumack BH, Aldrich FD. Toxicology of urea formaldehyde and polyurethane foam insulation. *JAMA*. 1981 Jan 16;245(3):243-3. DH499.

16. European Commission. Bisphenol-A: EU ban on baby bottles to enter into force tomorrow. Press release. 2011 May 31. DH489.

17. Needham LL. Exposure of the U.S. population to Bisphenol A and 4-tertiary-octylphenol: 2003-2004. *Environ Health Persp.* 2008 Jan;116(1):39-44. DH500.

18. Ibid.

19. Boas M, Main KM, Feldt-Rasmussen U. Environmental chemicals and thyroid function: an update. *Curr Opin Endocrinol Diabetes Obes.* 2009 Oct;16(5):385-91. DH501.

20. Wikipedia: Bisphenol A. Accessed 10/21/11. DH419.

21. Ibid.

22. Ibid.

23 Perera F, Vishnevetsky J, Herbstman JB, Calafat AM, Xiong W, Rauh V, Wang S. Prenatal bisphenol a exposure and child behavior in an inner-city cohort. *Environ Health Perspect.* 2012 Aug;120(8):1190-4. DH579.

24. Wikipedia: Coal tar. Accessed 2013 Jan. DH502.

25. Ibid.

26. Lambrozo J, Touitou Y, Dab W. Exploring the EMF-Melatonin Connection: A Review of the Possible Effects of 50/60-Hz Electric and Magnetic Fields on Melatonin Secretion. *Int J Occup Environ Health.* 1996 Jan;2(1):37-47. DH503.

27. Falzone N, Huyser C, Becker P, Leszczynski D, Franken DR. The effect of pulsed 900-MHz GSM mobile phone radiation on the acrosome reaction, head morphometry and zona binding of human spermatozoa. *Int J Androl.* 2011 Feb;34(1):20-6. DH504.

28. Franzellitti S, Valbonesi P, Ciancaglini N, Biondi C, Contin A, Bersani F, Fabbri E. Transient DNA damage induced by high-frequency electromagnetic fields (GSM 1.9 GHz) in the human trophoblast HTR-8/SVneo cell line evaluated with the alkaline comet assay. *Mutat Res.* 2010 Jan 5;683(1-2):35-42. DH96.

29. Divan HA, Kheifets L, Obel C, Olsen J. Cell phone use and behavioural problems in young children. *J Epidemiol Community Health.* 2012 Jun;66(6):524-9. DH505.

30. Dubey RB, Hanmandlu M, Gupta SK. Risk of brain tumors from wireless phone use. *J Comput Assist Tomogr.* 2010 Nov-Dec;34(6):799-807. DH506.

31. Volk HE, Lurmann F, Penfold B, Hertz-Picciotto I, McConnell R. Traffic-Related Air Pollution, Particulate Matter, and Autism. *AMA Psychiatry.* 2013;70(1):71-77. DH517.

32. Williams K, Helmer M, Duncan GW, Peat JK, Mellis CM, Perinatal and maternal risk factors for autism spectrum disorders in New South Wales, Australia. *Child Care Health Dev.* 2008 Mar;34(2):249-56. PMID:18257794. DH242.

33. Roberts JW, et al. Monitoring and reducing exposure of infants to pollutants in house dust. *Rev Environ Contam Toxicol.* 2009;201:1-39. DH268.

11

Heavy Metal Madness

Heavy metals are another category of toxic substances in our environment. Mercury, lead, cadmium, arsenic, antimony, and aluminum are toxic in even small amounts. These metals cause havoc in the body in a multitude of ways: they bind proteins needed for metabolism, they cause tissue damage, and they often produce a chronic cycle of oxidative stress and inflammation.

Acute toxicity from a large exposure to a heavy metal is uncommon. If a person knows they were exposed to a large amount of lead and become sick shortly afterwards, it is easy to correlate the illness with the exposure. Much more common (and more difficult to identify) is a chronic low dose exposure that causes many non-specific signs like fatigue, sadness, difficulty concentrating, depression, and anxiety. In the integrative medical community, the impact on health from low-dose chronic toxin exposure is well accepted. Since long-term exposure is difficult to measure and the symptoms are not unique to a specific metal, the traditional western medical system is slow to acknowledge the problem.

The list below shows the wide range of symptoms caused by these heavy metals. The symptoms also overlap, so it is difficult to tell just by symptoms which metal could have caused the problem. Looking into exposure history can help. Symptoms of heavy metal toxicity also overlap with symptoms of low thyroid function or low adrenal function, which makes sense because these metals can impair hormone function. They can also impair function of the female hormones, estrogen and progesterone, leading to problems with fertility.

Non-specific heavy metal symptoms

- Irritability
- Depression
- Difficulty concentrating
- Jumpiness/nervousness
- Poor memory
- Problems making decisions
- Numbness or tingling
- Decreased feeling in limbs
- Frequent insomnia
- Tremors
- Tics
- Burning tongue
- Ringing in the ears
- Twitching muscles
- Metallic taste in the mouth
- Constant itchy skin
- Unexplained skin rashes
- Diarrhea
- Constipation
- Bloating
- Frequent heartburn
- Headaches
- Leg cramps
- Constant pain in the joints

- High blood pressure
- Fast heart beat
- Cold hands/feet
- Chronic anemia
- Shortness of breath
- Chronic inflammation
- Fatigue

During pregnancy, the primary concern is the serious neurotoxic effects of heavy metals even in low doses.[1] An unborn child with a developing nervous system is especially vulnerable to these heavy metals. These metals readily pass through the placenta[2] and breast milk.[3,4] Mercury, lead, cadmium, and arsenic all bioconcentrate in the placenta. Therefore, an unborn infant could be exposed to an even higher level in the placenta than is present elsewhere in the pregnant woman.

Because of the serious concerns to an unborn infant from these metals, it is critical to address these issues before pregnancy. Avoiding these metals as much as possible is a good first step. Learning sources of heavy metals is important since many are found in unexpected places.

The next steps, described in later chapters, are to identify stored metals in the body and increase detoxification ability in the body. Again, it is only safe to detoxify *before* pregnancy!

Mercury

Mercury has been known for centuries to be dangerous to humans. The phrase "Mad as a hatter" refers to symptoms of mercury poisoning in people who used mercury in hat production.

Psychiatric and neurological effects of mercury include depression, irritability, anxiety, and seizure-like movements with strange limb shaking and unsteady gaits. Today we know not only that mercury is toxic, but also that the developing nervous system in fetuses and children is especially vulnerable. Mercury is stored in specific organs in the body, especially in the brain (leading to its severe neurological symptoms) and the kidneys.

Multiple symptoms can be seen from both acute and chronic mercury exposure. The scientific correlation between mercury and clinical symptoms has been from acute toxic exposures. One example from the 1950s was the development of Pink Disease in children from exposure to high levels of mercury from contaminated teething treatments and worm medicine. These children exhibited unusual behaviors such as retreating into their own worlds, difficulty with speech, and strange movements such as hand flapping and spinning.

Exposure to mercury comes from several known sources. The two primary sources today are from eating contaminated fish and from "silver" dental amalgams or fillings in the mouth. Methylmercury is the form found in fish.

Mercury in fish

The National Resources Defense Council (www.nrdc.org) has categorized fish species by their level of mercury. The NRDC also lists how much tuna a person can eat safely based on their weight, with specific caution for pregnant women and children. Since mercury is so toxic and dangerous to the developing brain, I recommend that women considering pregnancy only eat fish in the least mercury category. Salmon is in this safer category and it has healthy omega-3 fatty acids. However, when women are pregnant, I recommend they do not eat *any* seafood and to have only limited seafood when nursing. Omega-3 fats such as DHA are critically important but they can be obtained from high quality supplements checked to be free of mercury.

Mercury in your mouth

The other primary source of mercury comes from "silver" dental fillings or amalgams, which contain mercury. Actually, they don't just "contain" mercury; they consist of 50% mercury[5] and should be called "mercury fillings."

Concern has been raised about the use of mercury in dental amalgams since their development in the 1800s—even then it was known that mercury was toxic. Yet the practice of using silver amalgams (mercury fillings) became standard. These fillings are actually a composite of mercury with added silver, copper, and tin.[6] The form of mercury in the amalgams is inorganic mercury and it was thought to be inactive in the mouth. The problem is that the inorganic mercury is turned into methylmercury in the mouth and the intestines by bacteria. Methylmercury is known to be very toxic and is the form found in fish. Methylmercury easily crosses the placenta and the blood brain barrier, both of which are meant to protect an infant. Proof that mercury crosses into the brain comes from postmortem studies of people who had silver dental amalgams.[7]

The concentration of mercury in the brain correlates with the number of dental amalgams. People with silver dental amalgams have mercury levels 2 to 10 times higher than those without the amalgams.

In addition to being wrong about the inactivity of the mercury, amalgam proponents were also wrong in stating that older fillings emitted less mercury. Studies have documented mercury vapors coming from old silver amalgams.[8] These vapors are released regularly by everyday activities such as eating food, chewing gum, brushing teeth, and drinking hot liquids.

In my opinion, for maternal health there is no safe level of mercury exposure since it one of the most toxic substances to humans. However, according to the EPA, a "safe" exposure of mercury is 0.1 ug/kg (micrograms per kilogram of body weight) per day. It is estimated that a person with 1 to 4 amalgams is exposed to 8 ug/day. Exposure is increased with more amalgams. It is estimated that a person with 12 or more is exposed to 29 ug/day.

An average newborn at the time of delivery weighs about 7 to 8 lbs or roughly 3.5 kgs so a "safe" exposure would be 0.35 ug/day. If the pregnant woman has even 1 amalgam, the potential risk of exposure across the placenta before birth could be up to 8 ug/day, 22 times the recommended daily "safe" exposure. Research has shown as the number of amalgams a pregnant woman has increases, so does her risk of having a child with autism.[9]

Governments in Norway, Sweden, and Denmark have reviewed the health concerns about silver amalgams and have banned their use in dentistry. Other countries, such as Germany, France, Finland, Austria, and Canada have also taken cautionary stances and warned against their use in pregnant women. In the U.S., the FDA is currently assessing the health risks from these amalgams, although many dentists choose to no longer use them.

Luckily people in the U.S. are becoming more aware of the dangers of silver amalgams and are having them removed. It is very important to have them removed safely by a dentist trained in removal. The International Academy of Oral Medicine and Toxicology (www.iaomt.org) is the perfect place to look for a qualified dentist. Without the proper use of dental dams and suction devices, a person could get an increased acute dose of mercury during the removal process. Because of this risk, even with proper precautions, I would not recommend that women remove their silver dental amalgams during pregnancy or nursing. The ideal time would be several months before pregnancy so there would be adequate time for detoxification from any potential exposure.

Since mercury is a known neurotoxin and very dangerous to all growing children, removing dental amalgams before pregnancy is a crucial factor in avoiding autism and ADHD. The key point is to have them removed safely by a trained dentist with adequate time before the pregnancy to detoxify properly. Following amalgam removal, stored mercury in the body needs to be removed. There are products that absorb mercury in the intestine. Chlorella (a type of green algae) and zeolite (an absorbent blend of minerals) bind to mercury. Optimizing the detoxification pathways as described the Chapter 14 is also important.

Environmental mercury

Unfortunately, mercury is also in our environment: in our air, soil, and water. A primary environmental source is from coal burning plants. Even in my state of Colorado, which is a leader in researching green sources of energy, it has been challenging to wean off of coal. Forty-eight tons of mercury is still being pumped into our air each year from coal-fired power plants across the country.[10] The mercury in the air finds its way into soil, rivers, and oceans, and eventually contaminates our fish. While the U.S. is beginning to make environmental changes, unfortunately some countries such as China are increasing their coal burning with worldwide impacts.

A new source of mercury is the compact fluorescent light (CFL) bulbs, which are replacing incandescent bulbs in some countries. If a CFL bulb breaks, there is a large concern for acute mercury exposure. Think about having one of CFL bulbs break in a child's or pregnant woman's room and the subsequent dangerous release of mercury vapor. Cleanup of a broken CFL poses an additional exposure risk. Thermometers with mercury have been banned for this very reason, yet we have recently added a new fragile mercury source with similar health concerns.

Mercury in vaccines

The final source of mercury is the mercury preservative *thimerosal* that was used in many vaccines for children until 2001. Thimerosal is made from ethylmercury that was once thought to be safe in vaccines like inorganic mercury in dental amalgams. Yet for many years children would receive multiple doses of vaccines with thimerosal beginning at birth. Although thimerosal was not viewed to be dangerous to children by the traditional medical community, as a precaution it was taken out of most vaccines. Many vaccines contain a trace of thimerosal and whether this trace is dangerous is unknown. The influenza vaccine is available without thimerosal, however flu shots containing thimerosal are still given to children and pregnant women. If a person decides to receive a flu shot, they should select one that is preservative-free and without thimerosal.

Lead

Lead is another dangerous metal. This danger was recognized after children ingested lead paint. Although it was phased out several decades ago, lead paint is often present under newer paint in old houses. Anytime a window is opened, the friction of the window can aerosolize small particles of paint containing lead. These particles can also get in the soil and pollute the environment. Children then become exposed to lead by playing in the soil.

In addition to lead paint, leaded gasoline produces pollution that continues to be part of our ecosystem. Although cars do not use leaded gasoline anymore, it is still used in some farm machinery and boats. Coal burning plants are also an ongoing source of lead exposure (along with mercury). Many environmental groups are working to ban coal-produced energy in favor of cleaner, healthier energy sources.

Certain occupations may have increased lead exposure. Anyone working with paints or ceramics may be at risk since lead is used in glazes. Plumbers and electrical workers may also have exposure risk. Even supposedly "lead-free" brass fixtures can have a small amount of lead.

Recently lead has been found in a variety of unexpected places such as imported toys, medicines, and candy. Even some soft vinyl lunch-boxes have been found to contain lead.

Lead is stored in the nervous system, kidneys, and bones. This can contribute to a large range of symptoms such as headaches, dizziness, weight loss and abdominal pain. It also has significant effects on the cardiovascular system and is thought to be a contributor to heart disease and high blood pressure. Since lead is stored in bone, it leads to weaker bones and osteoporosis as people age.

For decades it has been known that lead is a neurotoxin and can reduce intelligence in developing children. Its effects on the nervous system result in problems with behavior and mental functioning. Children can also exhibit symptoms of ADHD and learning disorders from lead toxicity. These effects are compounded when an iron deficiency is present. If a child is iron deficient, they will have a greater absorption of lead.[11] When exposed to lead, children absorb up to 50%, compared to adults who may absorb only 10-15%.

Avoiding lead is key to neurological and behavioral health in children.

Cadmium

In terms of autism and ADHD neurotoxicity, most concerns have concentrated on mercury and lead. We need to remember that other heavy metals can also be neurotoxic and cause chronic disease. Even in small amounts, cadmium is a very toxic substance. Its toxicity is worsened when there is a deficiency of zinc, iron, and calcium. Zinc is protective from cadmium toxicity and as our diets are increasingly lower in zinc, we may begin to see more issues associated with cadmium exposure.

Cigarettes are high in cadmium and therefore smokers (and their children) are at increased risk. Quitting before pregnancy will dramatically reduce the risks from cadmium. Other sources include paints, food produced with contaminated fertilizer, water pipes, nickel/cadmium batteries, and electroplating.

Many of the symptoms of cadmium toxicity are similar to zinc deficiency. Cadmium replaces zinc in the body's chemical reaction binding sites. Some of these replacements cause neurotoxicity by interfering with neurotransmitters in the brain. We know about the importance of zinc for cognition and development so adequate zinc will help to protect from cadmium exposure.

Cadmium is stored primarily in the kidneys so it is a contributor to chronic kidney disease in adults with associated issues such as bone loss, anemia, and abnormal vitamin D production. It also appears that cadmium acts as an estrogen mimicker and can promote cancer[12] in both men and women.

Arsenic

Arsenic has been a known poison for centuries. Worldwide, arsenic levels have risen in water and food. Water contaminated with arsenic has created concerns about high arsenic levels in rice and other foods. In the U.S., arsenic is used as a growth promoter in non-organic chicken (another good reason to buy organic). Before regulations were put into place in 2003, arsenic was used as a preservative in wood for outdoor play equipment. Although this practice has been replaced, be wary of old decks and play sets as a source of exposure.

As a toxic substance, arsenic causes a multitude of problems. On a molecular level, it disrupts cellular mitochondrial energy formation and causes oxidative stress leading to inflammation. Arsenic toxicity is often first noted in the skin with darkening of the palms and soles with a subsequent increase in skin cancer risk. There is also a higher risk of lung and liver cancer.

Arsenic is neurotoxic for all ages. Research has found problems with neurodevelopment from early arsenic exposure. Adults are also at risk from ongoing exposure. Arsenic can lead to cognitive decline in older adults with a similar pattern to Alzheimer's disease.

Antimony

Antimony is a metal that is chemically similar to arsenic but less toxic. It is also found in cigarette smoke and gunpowder. Flame retardant clothing such as bedding and pajamas can be a source for women and children. Like arsenic, antimony disrupts the antioxidant system of glutathione in the body. In children, antimony may cause aggressive behavior.

Aluminum

Most people are exposed to aluminum on a daily basis. The primary exposure is from food including its use in preservatives, additives, food dyes, and baking powder. Other food-related exposure comes from aluminum pots/pans, aluminum foil, and aluminum cans. Aluminum contact with foods causes absorption of the metal. Tap water often contains aluminum. Fluoride in the water, especially if it is in the form of aluminum fluoride, increases our body's absorption of the aluminum. Several medicines contain aluminum, including specific antacids.

Cosmetics can be another source of daily exposure. Aluminum is a primary ingredient in most antiperspirants to help stop sweating. These underarm antiperspirants also contain toxic chemical parabens. Both of these chemicals are put under the arm where the drainage of the lymph system of the breast is located. Parabens are estrogen promoters and aluminum is an immune system stimulator. The combination may promote breast cancer.

Another method of aluminum exposure is its use in vaccines, which will be discussed in depth in Chapter 21. This exposure is different since the aluminum is injected directly into the body, as opposed to being ingested and processed by the digestive system.

How aluminum affects health

Aluminum targets three organ systems in the body. The first is the bones. Aluminum can be incorporated into the bone matrix leading to *osteomalacia* or weakening of the bones. The second system affected is the circulatory system: blood cells are altered leading to a type of anemia similar to anemia from iron deficiency. Finally, the third system affected is the neurologic system, especially the brain.

Since aluminum is stored in the brain, concern has been raised about its neurological and developmental effects. Aluminum crosses the placenta and can be passed through breast milk. Evidence of neurologic harm was first raised from a research study showing aluminum-induced nerve cell changes in the brain of patients with Alzheimer's disease. The same type of nerve cell changes in the brains of Alzheimer's patients has been found in children with autism.[13] This is extremely frightening. Alzheimer's is a chronic degenerative disease with deterioration of brain function and we are now finding similar changes in children with autism. It is remarkable that some children with developing nervous systems already have chronic inflammatory and degenerative changes in their brain cells. We know that aluminum causes inflammation because it is used in vaccines as a stimulator of the immune system. In fact, a 2012 study found that children with autism were especially vulnerable to aluminum in vaccines.[14] Aluminum is added so the body has a larger immune response, with the intent of having better protection from the vaccine. This is a double-edged sword that we need to understand more fully to gauge its impact on the body.

Summary

Just like the chemicals in our environment, heavy metals are part of our world. The madness in heavy metals arises when they are placed as ingredients in substances we use on a daily basis. We should not have to worry about exposure in food, dental fillings, air, soil and water, but we do. Awareness of where these metals hide is critically important for women contemplating pregnancy in order to avoid them as much as possible.

CHAPTER 11 REFERENCES

1. Amaya E, Gil F, Freire C, Olmedo P, Fernández-Rodríguez M, Fernández MF, Olea N. Placental concentrations of heavy metals in a mother-child cohort. *Environ Res.* 2013 Jan;120:63-70. DH515.

2. Autrup H. Transplacental transfer of genotoxins and transplacental carcinogenesis. *Environ Health Perspect.* 1993 Jul;101 Suppl 2:33-8. DH507.

3. Marques RC, Dórea JG, Bernardi JV, Bastos WR, Malm O. Prenatal and postnatal mercury exposure, breastfeeding and neurodevelopment during the first 5 years. *Cogn Behav Neurol.* 2009 Jun;22(2):134-41. DH423.

4. Schlunpf M, et al. Endocrine active UV filters: Developmental toxicity and exposure through breast milk. *Chimisa.* 2008b;62:1-7. DH272.

5. Wikipedia – Dental amalgam controversy. Accessed 10/21/11. DH26.

6. Ibid.

7. Nylander M, Friberg L, Lind B. Mercury concentrations in the human brain and kidneys in relation to exposure from dental amalgam fillings. *Swed Dent J.* 1987;11(5):179-87. DH508.

8. Ishitobi H, Stern S, Thurston SW, Zareba G, Langdon M, Gelein R, Weiss B. Organic and inorganic mercury in neonatal rat brain after prenatal exposure to methylmercury and mercury vapor. *Environ Health Perspect.* 2010 Feb;118(2):242-8. DH509.

9. Geier DA, Kern JK, Geier MR. A prospective study of prenatal mercury exposure from maternal dental amalgams and autism severity. *Acta Neurobiol Exp (Wars).* 2009;69(2):189-97. DH511.

10. Wright RO, Shannon MW, Wright RJ, Hu H. Association between iron deficiency and low-level lead poisoning in an urban primary care clinic. *Am J Public Health.* 1999 July; 89(7): 1049-53. DH513.

11. Ibid.

12. Siewit CL, Gengler B, Vegas E, Puckett R, Louie M. Cadmium Promotes Breast Cancer Cell Proliferation by Potentiating the Interaction between ER and c-Jun. *Mol Endocrinol.* 2010 May; 24(5): 981–992. DH514.

13. Vargas DL, Nascimbene C, Krishnan C, Zimmerman AW, Pardo CA. Neurological activation and neuroinflammation in the brain of patients with autism. *Ann Neurol.* 2005 Jan;57(1):67-81. DH178.

14. Seneff S, Davidson R, Liu J. Empirical Data Confirm Autism Symptoms Related to Aluminum and Acetaminophen Exposure. *Entropy.* 2012, 14(11), 2227-2253. DH516.

12

Toxic Beauty

On a typical day most women use soap, shampoo, and conditioner in their shower. This is often followed by makeup with foundation, blush, and mascara. On average, women use 12 cosmetic products a day containing approximately 126 different chemicals! What is the safety of these chemicals?

Just as women need to read the labels on food, they need to read the ingredient labels on cosmetics. Any product with chemicals applied to the skin can be absorbed into the body and cause health problems, just as any chemical eaten in food. These chemicals can be stored in the body and then passed to a baby through the placenta or breast milk.

Research studies have found multiple environmental chemicals in newborn cord blood, including those from cosmetics.[1] A newborn baby has not had a chance to use any soap or lotion, but already the baby has taken on stores of chemicals. The only possible source of these chemicals is from their mother.

The questions then become, which chemicals need to be avoided, and what are good alternatives? This chapter describes categories of the worst offenders. Two good sources for alternatives are *A Consumer's Dictionary of Cosmetic Ingredients* by Ruth Winter and the Environmental Working Group's Skin Deep Cosmetics Database http://www.cosmeticsdatabase.com.

Cosmetic Safety Regulations

The U.S. Food and Drug Administration (FDA) regulates cosmetics just as it regulates our food supply. Unfortunately the FDA has less control over cosmetics, and no authority to require cosmetic companies to do safety testing *before* the products are put on the market. Therefore, companies can put almost any chemical in a product and sell it with minimal or no safety testing. If problems are noted *after* the product is on the market, then more safety research can be done.

The cosmetic industry has a self-regulatory panel called the Cosmetics Ingredients Review (CIR). Since its inception more than 30 years ago, the CIR has only reviewed the safety of approximately 11% of the ingredients in cosmetics, and just nine ingredients were banned as unsafe. Considering there are more than 10,000 chemical ingredients in personal care products, the CIR has barely scratched the surface of ensuring our safety. This panel does not research combined chemicals, yet most women are putting products with multiple ingredients on their skin. Unfortunately, research on toxins and their effects on women, babies in utero, and young children is severely lacking.

The lax U.S. regulation is of more concern when we examine how other countries regulate this industry. Unlike the U.S., which bans chemicals *after* they have been used, the European Union (E.U.) uses a more preventative approach. An E.U. cosmetics directive bans many chemicals deemed unsafe; if the chemical causes any harm, it is barred from use in cosmetics. This directive has banned more than 1,000 products or approximately 10 times the number of similar products banned in the U.S. Canada also has a much stricter policy and has banned multiple chemicals that are frequently used in U.S. products.

For example, the antibacterial triclosan is one chemical banned in other countries, but still used in the U.S. Triclosan's chemical structure is similar to pesticides, such as dioxin, yet it is found in the majority of our antibacterial soaps and instant hand sanitizers. When exposed to chlorine in tap water triclosan produces chloroform, a carcinogenic compound.[2] In addition, triclosan may contribute to bacterial resistance. Although the FDA is investigating triclosan, the chemical is still being used every day by millions of pregnant women and children.

Several states have tried to bypass the lenient federal regulations and set up their own rules. In 2005, California passed a law requiring that cosmetics manufacturers "…list all cosmetic products that contain any ingredients known or suspected to cause cancer, birth defects, or other reproductive harm." Washington State has banned phthalates or plastic stabilizers (see below). Both of these are valiant attempts to protect people from toxins.

The "Polluting P's" Continued

Just as there are several "polluting P's" in our food (think pesticides) and our environment (think plastics), there are also many "polluting P's" in our cosmetic products.

Phthalates

Chemicals in the group called phthalates are used to soften plastics and to give beauty products the textures we like in nail polish and hairspray and the fragrances in perfume. Unfortunately, phthalates have also been used in baby care products and plastic toys, including ones that babies put in their mouths. Medical devices (such as intravenous bags), vinyl floors, and auto interiors (giving off a "new car smell,") are all made with phthalate chemicals.

Why the concern? Phthalates are endocrine disruptors; they affect hormones in the body, such as estrogen, and have an adverse effect on the reproductive system. Several studies have shown that women exposed to phthalates during pregnancy are more likely to have boys with abnormal development of the genitals.[3] Adult males receiving normal environmental exposure to phthalates were also found to have sperm damage. We have increasing rates of infertility and that may be part of the reason. Obviously both men and women considering having children should avoid these substances.

Relationship of phthalates to autism and ADHD

A relationship between phthalates and autism and other neurodevelopmental disorders has recently been raised by research studies. The higher a woman's exposure to phthalates during pregnancy, the higher her child's incidence of ADHD[4] and behavior/learning issues. A second study found that there was a strong association of levels of phthalates in children and ADHD.[5] A third study found that infants and toddlers living in homes with vinyl floors (which emit phthalates) are twice as likely to have autism five years later.[6] Findings from this last study were surprising because the researchers were not looking for environmental risk factors associated with autism.

Although the health risks of phthalates were beginning to be identified early in the 1990s, the FDA's initial response was that people's exposure to these chemicals was limited. However, the Environmental Working Group released a study in 2002[7] showing 70% of cosmetics contained phthalates. This prompted the *Campaign for Safe Cosmetics*, with the mission to raise awareness of the potential harm caused by phthalates. The next year, the E.U. banned cosmetics containing phthalates. Women of child-bearing years appear to have much higher concentrations of phthalates than other consumer groups, and the risk to these women and their children is too great to not ban these chemicals.

In the meantime, what can mothers-to-be do? Unfortunately, phthalates are not listed directly on the label of many products. The term "fragrance" is often used and should make people wary. Other phthalates are listed as abbreviations of their chemical names such as DEP (diethyl phthalate), DBP (dibutyl phthalate), DEHP (di[2-ethyl-hexyl] phthalate), BzBP (benzyl piperazine, a chemical related to pthalates), DINP (diisononyl phthalate), and DMP (dimethyl phthalate). If the true ingredient name is hidden or it is not pronounceable, the product should be avoided.

Parabens

Derived from petroleum, parabens are very common ingredients in many cosmetics and in some food products. Up to 90% of personal care products contain some form of parabens. Used as preservatives, they prolong the shelf life of many products by preventing the overgrowth of bacteria. When people were tested for paraben exposure, more than 90% tested positive, and women, starting as early as adolescence, had some of the highest exposure.[8]

Parabens are another group of chemicals that, like phthalates, are endocrine disruptors. Multiple studies have raised concerns about parabens' effects on the reproductive system;[9,10] they act like estrogen and can harm male development and function. Estrogenic effects in women are also a concern because of breast cancer promotion.

Many antiperspirants have parabens in addition to aluminum. These chemicals are placed under the arms, near the breast cells' lymph drainage. This area is where the majority of breast cancers begin. To compound the problem, many women shave under their arms and then put antiperspirants on every morning. Cut hair follicles, like cut skin, may increase the absorption of these toxins.

Relation of parabens to autism

Animal studies of parabens have shown negative effects on the development of the brain, nervous system and social behavior.[11] No studies have shown any effects on human development. There are no negative studies, just not enough research. We need to know more about the effects of parabens on the nervous system, just as we need to know more about the adverse effects of phthalates. In the meantime, I would not expose my future child to a class of chemicals that affects hormones and body development.

Parabens are easier to identify on labels because most of them have the word paraben in their title (methylparaben, ethylparaben, and butylparaben). Any ingredient that has p-hydroxybenzoic acid or parahydroxybenzoic acid also contains parabens. Natural cosmetic companies are developing healthier preservatives, so options exist. Again, Europe is ahead of us and has banned at least one type of paraben. Keep reading those labels.

Polyethylene glycol or "eth" ingredients

Polyethylene glycol or PEG is a petroleum-based product. The primary concern with this chemical, along with any chemical with "eth" in the name, such as sodium laureth sulfate, is the contaminant 1,4-dioxane. This contaminant appears in bath products. It supposedly can be removed during manufacturing, but it often is not. Because 1,4-dioxane is a contaminant, it is often not listed on the label; a woman needs to look for "PEG" or "eth" in the ingredient list.

The chemical 1,4-dioxane is a cancer promoter; it irritates the lungs and the skin.[12] There is also strong concern about toxicity to the kidneys and the nervous system. When a baby is developing, especially in utero, it is critical to avoid all neurotoxins or even potential neurotoxins. Unfortunately 1,4-dioxane was found in a lot of baby care and kids' bath products in lab testing done in 2007. The chemical is found on California's list of chemicals known to cause cancer or birth defects.

Other Toxic Ingredients

The list of chemicals to watch out for in cosmetics does not end with the Polluting P chemicals. Unfortunately there are some other serious offenders. Most of the toxic chemicals cause harm by disrupting hormones or promoting cancer or both. Many of these chemicals also cause damage to the nervous system, which is especially damaging for developing children.

Antibacterial products

As mentioned earlier, triclosan is an antibacterial compound used in soaps. It is also used in many consumer products including toys. Along with the problem of triclosan combining with chlorine to form chloroform,[13] its effects on hormones are a major concern for women considering pregnancy and having children. Triclosan appears to decrease the amount of thyroid hormone, our master regulating hormone, produced by the body. In other animal studies, triclosan has also been shown to affect the hormones estrogen and testosterone.[14]

Coal Tar and Dyes

Neither the words *coal* nor *tar* beckons you to place them on your skin, yet they are used in several cosmetic products. Interestingly enough, they are used in products for skin conditions such as psoriasis and hair conditions such as dandruff. Yet these products can cause multiple skin reactions and sensitivities. Natural treatments exist for these medical conditions, many including fragrant essential oils, so avoiding coal tar should be easy.

Coal tar can also be used to make dyes for products. Although I automatically thought all coal tar dyes would show up as a black pigment, they can also be transformed to shades of blue and green—colors that are used in oral care products such as toothpaste and mouthwash. According to the labels of these products, we are not supposed to swallow these products, but our mucus membranes are wonderful at absorbing chemicals (which is why sublingual medicines are very effective). Any color that does not look like a color found in nature probably is not and should not be ingested.

Ethanolamines: DEA (diethanolamine) and TEA (triethanolamine)

In cosmetics, ethanolamines are used as foaming agents and emulsifiers. Adjusting the pH of products is another one of their uses. Several concerns have been raised by research, however. Ethanolamines may be carcinogenic, and they also cause skin sensitivity, which is not helpful in a skincare product.

The primary concern is ethanolamines deplete choline in the body.[15] Choline is needed for brain development and is a critical component of the neurotransmitter acetylcholine. Ethanolamines also deplete metabolites of choline, which are critical for the detoxification pathway methylation. This pathway often does not work well in children with autism.[16]

Formaldehyde

When I think of formaldehyde, I remember the horrible smell in anatomy lab as a first-year medical student. Formaldehyde is a powerful preservative used to maintain human cadavers. It is also used in many construction materials such as plywood, paint, and paper. Because formaldehyde is a vapor, it becomes part of the air and a source of pollution.

When I discovered that this preservative was used in cosmetics and vaccines, I knew that something this strong did not belong on my face or injected into my child. Now investigating the multiple health risks of formaldehyde, I found out that my concerns were justified. Research has shown that formaldehyde promotes cancer in animals by damaging DNA and inhibiting its repair. Inhalation of this chemical often causes damage to the lungs, and contact with the skin causes irritation. It does not make sense to me that formaldehyde is used in cosmetics, which are applied to the skin.

161

From a child health perspective, the neurotoxic effects are frightening. Animal research studies have shown that exposure to formaldehyde decreases the number of nerve cells in the hippocampus,[17] changes neurotransmitters associated with behavior problems such as aggression,[18] and even decreases fertility.[19] Some adult animals develop neurologic disease many years after formaldehyde exposure during infancy.[20]

Use of formaldehyde in cosmetics has been banned in Japan and several countries in Europe. Canada has placed limits on its use in cosmetics. Avoiding this chemical in cosmetics, in the home, and workplace seems wise. I wonder if pregnant women working in labs with formaldehyde are warned of this danger.

Nail polish and remover

The smell upon walking into a nail salon is enough for most people to realize the multitude of chemicals that exist in nail products. Most nail polish contains dyes, polish hardeners (such as nitrocellulose), formaldehyde, solvents (such as toluene), and plasticizers (such as phthalates). Several of these chemicals are harmful when used alone, but when combined together, it is unknown how they interact, what other toxins are formed, and how they affect us. To remove the polish, we usually use polish remover containing acetone, which can act as a narcotic and cause symptoms of drunkenness. The unfortunate salon workers who are exposed to these chemicals for hours a day have shown multiple health concerns from skin rashes and respiratory abnormalities to an increased risk of miscarriage.

I recommend women either forgo nail polish from preconception through the end of breastfeeding or to use newly available safe nail polish with an alcohol-based, non-acetone remover.

Hair dyes

Most women and some men today use hair dyes. Just as nail polishes, hair dyes contain multiple concerning chemical combinations. Hair dyes contain ammonia, peroxide, p-phenylenediamine (PPD), coal tar dyes, DEA, polyethylene glycol, formaldehyde precursors, and lead, all of which are toxins that cause health problems. Healthier options are coming on the market, but we still have a ways to go.

The only woman I know who has never used hair dye or bleach is my mother. She doesn't wear any makeup either. Perhaps this is part of her good health in her 70s.

Skin lighteners

The primary ingredient in skin lighteners is *hydroquinone.* This chemical compound decreases the production of melanin, the substance that causes darkening in the skin. Multiple studies have shown that hydroquinone may cause genetic damage, resulting in cancers ranging from leukemias to thyroid, liver, and kidney tumors. This substance has been banned in Europe. The FDA acknowledges these health concerns (including cancer) and proposed a ban in 2006, but it continues to be available over-the-counter.

Heavy metal madness in makeup

As we have learned, heavy metals are potent neurotoxins and should be avoided as much as possible. They are damaging to all of us, but especially to infants and children whose brains are developing. You would never think of heavy metals as typical ingredients in makeup, but aluminum, lead, and mercury are found in multiple products. Lead is found in lip gloss, and mercury is found in mascara. Aluminum is a main ingredient in most antiperspirants. Fortunately, more and more companies are making it easier to find beauty products without harmful chemicals.

Sunscreens

Sunscreens deserve their own category because they are used frequently and many of their chemical ingredients present health concerns. Combining chemicals can alter their risks. Finally, the mechanism of how these ingredients protect from the sun is different. Since it is recommended that sunscreen be used daily, we need to know what is going on our skin as we step outside.

In 2012, the FDA put forth new sunscreen regulations. The regulations require ingredient information from manufactures and labeling changes. However, the regulations appear to do little to address the ingredients described below that threaten children's health. It is up to each individual to fully understand the issues involved and protect themselves. The Environmental Working Group has a great online sun-screen guide to help us.

UVA and UVB protection

There are two primary types of ultraviolet light from the sun: UVA and UVB rays. UVA are the Aging rays, and UVB are the Burning rays. The new FDA sunscreen regulations require manufactures to label their products if they protect from both UVA and UVB rays. It is important to use a sunscreen that contains both UVA and UVB coverage.

Types of sunscreens

Currently there are two classes of sunscreens, and they both carry health risks:

1. *Physical sunblock* contains zinc oxide and/or titanium oxide. Once placed on the skin, these chemicals block the sun's rays from reaching your skin.

2. *Chemical sunblock* works by being absorbed into the skin to stop the sun's rays from reaching the skin.

Health concerns for sunscreens

Nanoparticle toxicity

With physical sunscreens, the primary concern is the small size of zinc and titanium particles (called *nanoparticles*). We all probably remember the complete white coat of zinc oxide cream on the skin of lifeguards. With the advent of nanoparticles, however, zinc oxide can now be rubbed into the skin and not seen. Manufacturers claim that nanoparticles provide a physical block without being absorbed in the skin. But studies have shown absorption into both intact and damaged skin.[21,22] In fact, nanoparticles are being studied as a delivery method for transdermal (on the skin) medications. If nanoparticles are not ab-sorbed into the skin, it would make no sense for them to be used to help a medication get through the skin into the body.

Research has also shown toxicity inside of cells caused by nanopar-ticles of titanium in sunscreen.[23] Any substance that has the potential to enter cells and change the structure inside the cell has the potential to disrupt DNA. Disrupted DNA definitely contributes to the develop-ment of cancer.

Toxic metals

Although both zinc and titanium are used in sunscreens, there is a difference between the two substances. Zinc is an essential mineral that is often low in diets and very low in children with autism. On the other hand, titanium is a toxic metal, and we don't know the long-term effects of titanium on the body. I have often seen elevated titanium levels in children with autism. Titanium is also a very allergenic metal, similar to nickel, that causes skin rashes.

Hormone disruptors

The primary concern of sunscreens is that they contain hormone disruptors. Yes, another chemical that we put on our bodies and therefore into our bodies that causes hormone disruption! One study found concern for endocrine effects on human health from UV chemical sunscreens.[24] Mammal research into UV filters has also shown potential exposure in utero, resulting in delayed male puberty and reduced weight of reproductive organs based on the amount of exposure.[25]

Free radicals

Sunscreens stop UVB radiation, which stops sunburn, and this is where the skin protection factor (SPF) rating comes in. However, UV radiation from the sun also generates free radicals. Free radicals are an important part of protecting cells, but an excess of them can kill cells.

Sunscreen manufacturers know about the free radical formation, and they add antioxidants to their products to combat this problem. When people do not use sunscreens correctly, such as not reapplying the sunscreen correctly or not using enough, which commonly happens, the free radical protection is very low.

Vitamin D blockers

Vitamin D is of critical importance to very many functions of the body and there are vitamin D receptors on every cell in the body. It is necessary for bone growth, calcium absorption, immune function, cancer prevention, blood sugar control, gene regulation, and mood stabilization, to name just a few benefits. Our primary source of vitamin D is from the sun, not from food. Because sunscreens block our ability to make vitamin D in the skin, levels of this important vitamin have been decreasing in all populations studied, including children and pregnant women. This is concerning, especially given vitamin D's significant health benefits.

To ensure natural vitamin D production, I recommend brief early morning sun exposure to as much of the body as possible for no more than 15 minutes, while wearing a hat to limit sun exposure to the face.

Options for sun safety

Public health agencies recommend skin coverage and timing as good first-line precautions from sun damage: coverage of the skin with protective clothing, shade protection, and avoiding the strong midday sun.

The recommended second line defense is sunscreen. I only recommend sunscreen products with zinc oxide.

Labeling

Labeling of cosmetics should be changed to avoid confusion from marketing terms such as "natural," "green," "organic," and "dermatologist-tested." These words are commonly used on packaging to make the products appear healthy and entice consumers to buy them. However, these marketing terms do not guarantee that harmful chemicals are not present. "Natural" can include anything found in nature (petroleum) or metals (aluminum or lead).

"Green" products are the current fad. While the word *green* is supposed to imply that a product is good for the environment, the term does not necessarily mean it is healthy. A product with a green label may mean this product is better than other products for the environment, although both may be toxic to an individual. *Organic* is another confusing term. Technically it means something that contains carbon, but concerning food and ingredients, organic means something not produced with pesticides. Be wary also of products that list "fragrance," even "natural fragrance." "Dermatologist-tested" is another confusing term used to imply safety. Many dermatologists recommend prescription medicines and products to their patients because they might clear up skin rashes. However, prescription products may contain chemicals that will cause internal health or long-term health problems.

Cosmetic Options

Less is better. Fewer products and fewer ingredients are usually healthier. A simple basic soap, such as unscented glycerin soap, and a single oil, or moisturizing lotion, such as sweet almond oil or shea butter, covers most needs. Choosing a deodorant without aluminum and preservatives is a big safety improvement. Finally, women should buy cosmetics and personal care items from a company that lists both what they have and do not have in their products. If the manufacturer lists all of their ingredients, they likely know the dangerous chemicals to exclude, and they are letting you know that they have done the research to make a safer product.

Summary

Our environment today is loaded with chemicals. Most of them have not been adequately tested for safety in women and children. Any chemical that a woman is exposed to can be passed to her infant during pregnancy and nursing. This exposure comes at a crucial time in a vulnerable developing child. There is no question in my mind and in the minds of many others that the increasing amount of foreign toxic exposures is negatively impacting the health of our children.

The key for any woman contemplating pregnancy is to clean up her environment. She should look closely at all sources of potential exposures.

In the 1960s, Rachel Carson warned of the harm of chemicals to animals and plants in her groundbreaking book *Silent Spring*. It amazing me that she had so much foresight to predict the problems from these chemicals. It further astonishes me that we were unable to listen. Now we have not only hurt our wildlife, leading to a silent spring, but we have hurt our children. We now have silent children: the children with autism who are unable to speak, from an ignored silent spring written over 50 years ago.

CHAPTER 12 REFERENCES

1. Executive Summary, Environmental Working Group. Body Burden-The Pollution in Newborns: A benchmark investigation of industrial chemicals, pollutants, and pesticides in umbilical cord blood. *Environmental Working Group.* July 14, 2005. DH289.

2. Rule KL, Ebbett VR, Vikesland PJ. Formation of chloroform and chlorinated organics by free-chlorine-mediated oxidation of triclosan. *Environ Sci Technol.* 2005 May 1;39(9):3176-85. DH519.

3. Barrett JR. Phthalates and Baby Boys: Potential Disruption of Human Genital Development. *Environ Health Perspect.* 2005 August; 113(8): A542. DH520.

4. Engel SM, Miodovnik A, Canfield RL, Zhu C, Silva MJ, Calafat AM, Wolff MS. Prenatal Phthalate Exposure is Associated with Childhood Behavior and Executive Functioning. *Environ Health Perspect.* 2010 Jan 8. DH251.

5. Kim BN, et al. Phthalates exposure and attention-deficit/hyperactivity disorder in school-age children. *Biol Psychiatry.* 2009 Nov 15;66(10):958-63. DH262.

6. Ibid.

7. Environmental Working Group. Not too pretty – phthalates, beauty products and the FDA. 2002. DH518.

8. Calafat AM, Ye X, Wong LY, Bishop AM, Needham LL. Urinary concentrations of four parabens in the U.S. population: 2005-2006. *Env Health Persp.* 2010 May;118(5):679-85. DH339.

9. Kawaquichi M, Kawaguchi M, Morohoshi K, Imai H, Kato N, Himi T. Maternal exposure to isobutyl-paraben impairs social recognition in adult female rats. *Exp Anim.* 2010;59(5):631-5. DH261.

10. Chen J, Ahn KC, Gee NA, Gee SJ, Hammock BD, Lasley BL. Antiandrogenic properties of parabens and other phenolic containing small molecules in personal care products. *Toxicol Appl Pharmacol.* 2007 Jun 15;221(3):278-84. DH340.

11. Kawaquichi 2010.

12. Sarantis H, Malkan S, Archer L. Children's Bath Products Contaminated with Formaldehyde, 1,4-Dioxane. *Campaign for Safe Cosmetics.* 2009. DH492.

13. Rule KL, Ebbett VR, Vikesland PJ. Formation of chloroform and chlorinated organics by free-chlorine-mediated oxidation of triclosan. *Environ Sci Technol.* 2005 May 1;39(9):3176-85. DH519.

14. Triclosan, Wikipedia, accessed Aug 2010. DH274.

15. Diethanolamine, Wikipedia, accessed Aug 2010. DH249.

16. James SJ, Cutler P, Melnyk S, Jernigan S, Janak L, Gaylor DW, Neubrander JA. Metabolic biomarkers of increased oxidative stress and impaired methylation capacity in children with autism. *Am J Clin Nutr.* 2004;80(6):1611-1617. DH296.

17. Sarsilmaz M, Kaplan S, Songur A, Colakoglu S, Aslan H, Tunc AT, Ozon OA, Turgut M, Bas O. Effects of postnatal formaldehyde exposure on pyramidal cell number, volume of cell layer in hippocampus and hemisphere in the rat: a stereological study. *Brain Res.* 2007 May 11;1145-67. DH357.

18. Liu Y, Ye Z, Luo H, Sun M, Li M, Fan D, Chui D. Inhalative formaldehyde exposure enhances aggressive behavior and disturbs monoamines in frontal cortex synaptosome of male rates. *Neurosci Lett.* 2009 Oct 23;464(2):113-6. DH359.

19. Taskinen HK, Kyyronen P, Sallmen M, Vertanen SV, Liukkonen TA, Huida O, Lindbohm ML, Anttila A. Reduced fertility among female wood workers exposed to formaldehyde. *Am J Ind Med.* 1999 Jul;36(1):206-12. DH355.

20. Songur A, Ozen AA, Sarsilmaz M. The toxic effects of formaldehyde on the nervous system. *Rev Environ Contam Toxicol.* 2010;203:105-18. DH356.

21. Gulson B, et al. Small amounts of zinc from zinc oxide particles in sunscreens applied outdoors are absorbed through human skin. *Toxicol Sci.* 2010 Aug 12. DH257.

22. Jiang R, Roberts MS, Collins DM, Benson HA. Absorption of sunscreens across human skin: an evaluation of commercial products for children and adults. *British Journal of Clinical Pharmacology.* 48(4): 635-37. DH260.

23. Choksi AN, Poonawalla T, Wilkerson MG. Nanoparticles: a closer look at their dermal effects. *J Drugs Dermatol.* 2010 May;9(5):475-81. DH247.

24. Schlumpf M, Cotton B, Conscience M, Hller V, Steinmann B, Lichtensteiger W. In vitro and in vivo estrogenicity of UV screens. *Environ Health Perspect.* 2001 Mar;109(3):239-44. DH270.

25. Schlumpf M, et al. Endocrine activity and developmental toxicity of cosmetic UV filter—an update. *Toxicology.* 2004 Dec 1;205(1-2):113-22. DH271.

13

Building a Strong Detoxification System

After learning about the multitude of toxins in our environment, I hope it is evident that women need to detoxify their bodies before getting pregnant. It is impossible to prevent all exposure to toxic chemicals in today's world. Education and avoidance of toxins are imperative for improving health.

The next strategy is to strengthen the body's natural ability to detoxify. This is largely done through improving the biochemistry of the liver and kidneys. The goal is to make metabolism work better by giving it the specific building blocks it needs to function properly. The following chapter describes the last step for avoiding toxin heath risks: safe practices for removing chemicals.

Before pregnancy is a critically important time to remove toxins that have accumulated in the woman to improve her chances of having a healthy baby. Changes to diet and digestive support, while optimally started before pregnancy, are still safe to implement during pregnancy. However, detoxification is only safe before pregnancy. This is a point that has to be taken very seriously. Mobilizing toxins and removing them from the body has the potential to increase exposure to a child in utero or to a breastfed child.

Detoxification Organs

The liver is the primary organ of detoxification. It processes both toxins acquired from outside the body, and normal chemical breakdown products inside the body. The kidneys, lungs, intestines, and skin are also important detoxifying organs. Toxins enter the body primarily through ingestion. Inhalation and skin contact are other normal routes. From these entry points, chemicals are then transported directly to the liver, where the biochemical detoxification takes place. The substances are then removed from the body by transfer to the intestines or kidneys.

Biochemistry of Detoxification

There are two biochemical steps in detoxification of compounds: *phase 1* and *phase 2*. They need to be in balance for proper detoxification.

Phase 1 involves enzymes called *cytochrome P450 enzymes*. The highest concentration of cytochrome P450 enzymes is in the liver; lesser amounts are in the lungs and the kidneys. In phase 1 detoxification, toxins are chemically modified to a fat–soluble form to get them ready for the phase 2 reaction. After being metabolized by the phase 1 reactions, some chemicals actually become more toxic.

In phase 2 of the detoxification cycle, enzymes add a chemical compound to the modified toxin to form a water-soluble molecule— a process called *conjugation*. The water-soluble form of the toxin can then be easily passed out of the body through the kidneys or the intestine. There are several different kinds of conjugation during phase 2: acetylation, glucuronidation, amino acid conjugation (often with the amino acid glycine), glutathione conjugation, methylation, and sulfation. Different nutrients and supplements support different conjugation pathways.

If phase 2 detoxification does not work properly to change phase 1 intermediate chemicals, free radicals are produced. These free radicals contribute to toxicity and can lead to inflammation.

Genetic Individuality of Detoxification

There is a large variability in people's detoxification capacity. This can be explained in part by genetics. This is why some people have more side effects from medicines since they cannot detoxify them as well as others. It also explains why some people have fewer medical problems than others when exposed to the same toxin. In children with autism, research has found that many of these children have high toxic burdens[1] and genetic weaknesses in the ability to detoxify.[2,3,4] Thus, they have more problems from exposure to environmental toxins. Since this is genetic, many parents of children with autism also have genetic weaknesses in their ability to process toxins. They need to avoid toxins and to be careful when detoxifying.

In phase 1 detoxification, there are at least 50 different cytochrome P450 enzymes. These 50 enzymes are controlled by 35 different genes. Each gene has two copies—one from the mother and one from the father. There are different forms of the genes called *genetic polymorphisms*. Some forms make the enzyme work faster so that a person is better at detoxifying, and some do the opposite. Research has shown that differences in genes can lead to wide variability in the cytochrome P450 enzyme capability even in healthy individuals.[5]

In phase 2 detoxification, there is also enzyme genetic variability from genetic polymorphisms.[6] This is the case with methylation in children with autism. They often have polymorphisms in the MTHFR gene that causes them to need more vitamin B12 and special forms of folate.[7] This polymorphism decreases their ability to detoxify many compounds, including neurotransmitters.

Since there can be genetic variability in both phase 1 and 2, these two systems can get out of balance. If the phase 1 system is more active, an increase in toxic free radicals can accumulate which can cause increased inflammation. Increased phase 1 activity also produces increased symptoms associated with nervous, immune, and endocrine system diseases, and this is certainly true in autism. Increased phase 1 activity can also cause depletion of glutathione, which is one of the most prevalent antioxidants in the body and is often depleted in those with autism.[8]

Evaluation of the Detoxification System

There are specific tests that evaluate phase 1 and phase 2 detoxification processes. Phase 1 can be measured by a caffeine metabolism test. A specific amount of caffeine is given and then two saliva samples are taken. How quickly the caffeine is cleared gives information on how well the cytochrome P450 enzymes work. A slow caffeine clearance shows decreased activity of this enzyme and greater difficulty eliminating toxins. Even without doing this specific test most people have a rough idea about how they metabolize caffeine. There are those people who have a cup of coffee and are jumpy for hours and probably have decreased function of the phase 1 enzymes. The people that have good phase 1 function can drink a cup of coffee in the evening and fall asleep an hour later.

General phase 2 detoxification can be evaluated by the ingestion of acetaminophen (Tylenol™) and aspirin. This will give an overall indication of how well the phase 2 detoxification works by measuring breakdown of these substances in the urine.

Individual phase 2 enzyme genetic polymorphisms, such as those in the methylation pathway, can also be evaluated. The genetic polymorphism called MTHFR, that relates to the metabolism of vitamin B12 and folic acid, is most commonly evaluated. Genetic polymorphisms also exist for other enzymes, such as the enzymes that metabolize glutathione: the glutathione S-transferases. These enzymes help eliminate heavy metals such as mercury from the body and are often weak in some children with autism.[9] Test panels of genetic polymorphisms are available from specialized labs.

It is also important to determine whether phase 1 and phase 2 are in balance. Finding an imbalance would lead to treatments that support one phase more than the other.

Women with a history of liver and kidney disease or those who have been on multiple medicines should have a basic blood screening of liver and kidney function. There are liver function tests (ALT or alanine aminotransferase, AST or aspartate aminotransferase, bilirubin, and alkaline phosphatase) and kidney function tests (BUN and creatinine). All of these tests will return normal results unless there is some significant damage to either the liver or kidneys. Suboptimal function of these organs, however, is not normally determined by these tests.

Strengthening the Detoxification System

Certain nutrients must work well to support the detoxification organs and to strengthen each enzyme in the system. Those people with genetic polymorphisms may require more of certain nutrients or special, more active forms of certain nutrients, such as methyl B12 for methylation weaknesses.

Step 1: Improve diet

An organic diet as discussed in previous chapters goes a long way toward improving detoxification pathways. It eliminates a whole category of toxins by avoiding pesticides. Organic food typically contains more nutrients, so it will support overall nutrition.

Detoxification is impaired by insufficient calories and protein. Protein stores are important for the production of enzymes, amino acids, and peptides—all essential ingredients in the biochemical steps of detoxification. The enzymes in this process can also be poisoned by toxins such as heavy metals. The system can also be overwhelmed by too many toxins at the same time or from toxins that compete for the same detoxification pathway.

Step 2: Supplement with drainage or terrain formulas

Drainage, or terrain, formulas are primarily homeopathic and herbal products that help the process of detoxification. The nutrients for phase 1 and 2 detoxification help the biochemistry and the drainage formulas support the organs of elimination for the toxins. Therefore it is important to use separate remedies for the liver, kidney, and lymph system. Many practitioners recommend that a person begin with these remedies first and then add the nutrients to support detoxification later.

Step 3: Increase needed nutrients

The following key vitamins and minerals are needed to support detoxification:

Nutrients to support phase 1

- Minerals: calcium, iron, magnesium, molybdenum, selenium, and zinc
- Vitamins: A, B3, B6, B12, C, D3, E, and folic acid
- Supportive nutrients: N-acetyl cysteine, milk thistle (herb), citrus bioflavonoids, and quercetin

Nutirents to support phase 2

- Minerals: molybdenum and calcium D-glucarate (important for glucuronidation and hormone metabolism—often found in cruciferous vegetables such as broccoli and in fruits such as grapes, and apples)
- Vitamins: B1, B5, B12, C, choline, and folic acid
- Amino acids: L-carnitine, glutamine, glycine, lysine, methionine, and taurine
- Supportive nutrients: cruciferous vegetables, glutathione, milk thistle, MSM (sulfur compound), N-acetyl cysteine, and phytonutrients

Combination Products for Strengthening the Detoxification System

A good way to obtain the extra nutrients for a detoxification program is through a formula that supports both the phase 1 and phase 2 cycles. Multiple nutraceutical companies make these products, usually in a powder form with a type of protein. Most of these products come with detoxification plans including healthy diet recommendations such as lowering sugar intake, and increasing fruits and vegetables. If some of the above nutrients are needed for a particular woman, they can be found on the list of ingredients. A product label will often state that it promotes a certain aspect of detoxification such as improving liver function or supporting phase 1/phase 2 detoxification.

Individual Products for the Detoxification System

If a person is not interested in a combination product for detoxification, individual products can be combined. Important nutrients to include are those that promote glutathione formation and methylation.

If there are specific genetic polymorphisms, supplements need to be added to focus on these weak areas of detoxification.

I first recommend adding nutrients for methylation. Vitamin B12 and folic acid (both in the methyl form) are essential. Testing homocysteine levels are helpful as I described in Chapter 6, because if the level is above 6, there is a need for more of these vitamins. Methylation also requires a good source of protein since there are several amino acids that are critical for the process, such as methionine.

A source of glutathione is also important since it is the major antioxidant in the body. It is depleted quickly with increased exposure to toxins and stress. Cigarette smoking with its multiple toxins creating free radicals causes a large depletion in glutathione and vitamin C.

The primary problem with oral glutathione is that it is quickly changed to a form that cannot be used to help detoxification. Many forms found in health food stores will not help build the correct form of glutathione. There are two specific oral forms of glutathione that can be used. One is *liposomal glutathione* where the glutathione is enclosed in a fat molecule to help absorption. *Acetyl-glutathione* is also a good option.

Glutathione is naturally made in the body, so supplementing precursors or nutrients needed to form glutathione is another method of improving levels. *N-acetyl-cysteine* is one of the precursors of glutathione and is more stable and easily absorbed by mouth. Vitamin C and the herb milk thistle also help build glutathione and can be used with glutathione or N-acetyl-cysteine.

Glutathione is very effective if used by an intravenous or IV form, although obviously this is not practical for most people. For anyone with a serious chronic disease who is contemplating pregnancy, it may be good to contact a practitioner to discuss IV glutathione. Topical creams of both glutathione and N-acetyl-cysteine are available by prescription from compounding pharmacies. Inhaled glutathione is also available by prescription and is especially good for smokers and anyone with chronic lung disease.

When building glutathione or glutathione precursors, it is good to add supplements that help the glutathione work well. Often these are anti-oxidant formulas that contain extracts of fruits and vegetables called *phytonutrients*. One type of formula contains cruciferous vegetables, such as broccoli, that has the phytonutrient sulforophane. Polyphenolic compounds, such as pomegranate or pine bark extract, are other blends of phytonutrients. The complete detoxification products often contain several of these compounds.

Detoxification Supplements Summary

Combination detoxification products
Drainage or terrain formulas
- or -
Individual products including:

- Adequate protein
- Methyl B12
- Methylfolate or folinic acid
- Vitamin B-complex or multi-vitamin
- Vitamin C
- Glutathione or its precursor N-acetylcysteine
- Anti-oxidant phytonutrient blend
- Drainage or terrain formulas

Summary

The purpose of building a strong detoxification system is two-fold: first, it strengthens the ability of the body to rid itself of ongoing day-to-day toxin exposure, and second, it helps eliminate some of the existing toxins that have been accumulated over the years without having to do further detoxification. By giving the body the necessary ingredients for the detoxification process, some toxins will be eliminated on their own.

If the detoxification system in the body is not working well, then detoxification may only move toxins around the body and not eliminate them. This is often why people may feel sick when they detoxify. Their body is not able to eliminate toxins. Thus it is important that women adequately prepare their bodies before they detoxify.

A combination of building the system and detoxifying the system is important for most people. It is critical for those with serious chronic illnesses before pregnancy.

Most people will need individualized guidance from an integrative practitioner experienced in detoxification for effective treatment.

CHAPTER 13 REFERENCES

1. Adams JB, Baral M, Geis E, Mitchell J, Ingram J, Hensley A, Zappia I, Newmark S, Newmark S, Gehn E, Rubin RA, Mitchell K, Bradstreet J, El-Dahr JM. The Severity of autism is associated with toxic metal body burden and red blood cell glutathione levels. *J of Toxicology.* 2009: ID 532640. DH521.

2. Currenti SA. Understanding and determining the etiology of autism. *Cell Mol Neurobiol.* 2010;30:161-171. DH107.

3. DeSoto C. Ockham's Razor and autism: the case for developmental neurotoxins contributing to a disease of neurodevelopment. *NeuroToxicology.* 2009;30:331-337. DH108.

4. Edwards TM, Myers JP. Environmental exposures and gene regulation in disease etiology. *Environ Health Perspect.* 2007;115(9):1264-1270. DH111.

5. Waring R, Emery P. The genetic origin of responses to drugs. *Br Med Bull.* 1995;51:449-61. DH580.

6. Ibid.

7. James SJ, et al. Metabolic endophenotype and related genotypes are associated with oxidative stress in children with autism. *Am J Med Genet B Neuropsychiatry Genet.* 2006;141B(8):947-956. DH296.

8. Rose S, Melnyk S, Pavliv O, Bai S, Nick TG, Frye RE, James SJ. Evidence of oxidative damage and inflammation associated with low glutathione redox status in the autism brain. *Transl Psychiatry.* 2012 Jul 10;2:e134. DH524.

9. Serajee FJ, Nabi R, Zhong H, Huq M. Polymorphisms in xenobiotic metabolism genes and autism. *J Child Neurol.* 2004 Jun;19(6):413-7. DH525.

14

Detoxification

Before a woman considers pregnancy it is important to figure out what toxins are present. Some toxins are more dangerous than others so a smaller amount of one toxin may be more harmful than a larger amount of another toxin. As discussed in previous chapters, especially concerning are the toxins that can cause problems in pregnancy, or harm a child's development. These include heavy metals such as mercury and lead which can harm a child's neurological development. Pesticides such as organophosphates that are used on yards and on non-organic food products are also harmful to a developing baby. Both heavy metals and pesticides are also a concern in the development of autism. It is also especially important to consider chemicals such as phthalates, which can cause birth defects.

Most women need some detoxification, especially going into a pregnancy. The length of the detoxification process depends on a person's health. For people who are healthy, a month-long detoxification plan with a detoxification formula and some positive diet changes may be enough. A sauna protocol or a homeopathic detoxification product may be very helpful.

For those with common toxicity symptoms, it is important to have a more thorough evaluation of toxins and a longer treatment protocol. Depending on symptoms, anywhere from six months to a year may be needed. Although this may sound like a long time period, the positive impact on health for both the mother and future child may be immense.

Common toxicity symptoms

- Headaches
- Fatigue
- Mucus congestion in nose, throat, and lungs
- Chronic joint and muscle aches
- Digestive problems such as irritable bowel syndrome
- Allergy symptoms such as irritated eyes, sneezing or congestion
- Environmental sensitivities to chemicals such as gasoline, perfumes or air fresheners
- Immune weakness (frequent or long-lasting infections)
- Mood issues such as depression and anxiety
- Sleep problems
- Skin rashes such as hives
- Decreased appetite
- Sore throat

Detoxification Help and Plan

For women experiencing multiple toxin symptoms, I strongly recommend that they meet with a practitioner experienced in toxin effects, testing, evaluation, and detoxification. The practitioner will review the symptoms and patient history. They often will recommend a detoxification protocol with supplemental detoxification formulas, and a healthy organic diet with high intakes of fruits, vegetables and adequate protein. An infrared sauna protocol (described below) may also be prescribed.

Fathers-to-be also need to detoxify. Their toxicity level affects their fertility, sperm count, and the future baby's health.

Toxin Testing and Evaluation

Once toxins get into the body, the body tries to clear them through detoxification pathways. If there are too many toxins, the body stores them in tissues. These tissues can be in any organ in the body but certain toxins tend to be stored in certain organs. For example, lead is often stored in bone. Fat-soluble toxins such as pesticides are stored in our fat cells.

To maximize health and address toxicity issues before pregnancy, we need to identify and measure toxins stored in the body. Since toxins are stored in tissues, ideally we would take samples of the particular tissues where the toxins are stored. Unfortunately this is impractical for most tissues such as bones or fat tissue.

An easy tissue to evaluate is hair. Hair tests give good information about minerals (e.g. zinc and calcium) and heavy metals. But they need to be conducted by reliable labs and interpreted by an experienced practitioner. In most cases, someone with a higher amount of a heavy metal such as mercury will indeed have a higher level on their hair test. The exception is someone with a very poor detoxification system. Their body has such difficulty eliminating toxins that they are not even seen in a hair sample. The heavy metal is stored in the organs, but the body cannot eliminate the metal well enough to be seen in the hair sample. This is often seen in children with autism who have a positive history of exposure to mercury but not a positive result on a hair test. The difficulty in interpreting hair tests has led some to question their use in practice. For an experienced practitioner, they are the easiest and cheapest way to obtain some preliminary information about heavy metals.

Blood is another tissue where toxins can be measured. The problem is that the body tries to get the toxins out of the blood quickly, so often the results from the blood test are normal. If a person experiences a large toxin exposure, a prompt blood test will show elevated toxin levels. However, if the test is given several days after the exposure, a toxin blood level may be normal because the toxin was already removed from the blood (but is still in the organs). The blood test may also show normal for long-term, low-level exposures. Some blood labs have more sensitive tests that can measure metals in smaller amounts. Some specialized laboratories can even measure metals inside red blood cells.

A red blood cell metal test has a better approximation of metals in the body than a general plasma blood test.

Since toxins are not easily measured in most tissues, many health care practitioners will measure toxins as they are removed from the body. Toxins are primarily removed through the digestive tract as stool or through the kidneys as urine. Since most exposures are low level, the toxin amounts in urine or stool would normally be too small to measure. Therefore practitioners will often do a "challenge test." Prior to this test, it is critically important that the detoxification system be strengthened.

In the challenge test, a person is given a substance that binds the toxin to bring it out of the body. Then the toxin level is measured in urine or stool. A higher amount of toxin that is eliminated indicates that a higher amount exists in the body. The challenge test is mainly done for heavy metals such as mercury and lead.

Toxicity

All of the above tests measure *exposure* to toxins such as heavy metals. *Toxicity* is defined as the negative health effects resulting from exposure to a toxin. Toxicity is more difficult to evaluate than exposure. For example, if the hair test or the urine "challenge" test shows mercury, we know that a person has been exposed to, or come into contact with mercury at some point in their life. It does not specifically tell us that this mercury has caused harm in the body or illness in the body, which is the argument used by traditional medicine not to treat environmental illness.

Other Testing

For toxins other than the heavy metals, an environmental pollutant test panel can be done from a urine sample. This panel measures harmful chemicals from our day-to-day environment such as phthalates, parabens, and styrene. These tests will determine if a mother-to-be has high levels of toxins linked to birth defects, developmental issues, and autism and ADHD. The important toxins to evaluate are the chemicals with the highest levels and the ones most harmful to a pregnant mother or young child, such as phthalates.

Toxin Evaluation Summary

Primary tests

- Hair - heavy metals
- Urine - environmental pollutants

Secondary tests (depending on personal history of illness or exposure):

- Urine - challenge test
- Blood, urine, and hair—complete mercury analysis

Infrared Sauna

An infrared sauna is different from those normally in health clubs because it penetrates further to remove more toxins but at a lower and safer temperature. The infrared sauna operates at less than 130 degrees while many regular saunas range from 160 to 200 degrees. Infrared is a band of the light spectrum that is not visible to the human eye, but can be felt as heat. Infrared heat is able to penetrate 1.5 to 2 inches deep into the body. This type of heat is very safe, is normally produced by our body tissues, and is used by the body for many healing purposes. The infrared sauna duplicates this heat and the tissues in our body absorb this heat, causing the water in the cell to react in a process called *resonant absorption*. This resonant absorption occurs when the infrared frequency matches the frequency of the water in the cell, causing toxins to be dropped off into the blood stream and excreted in sweat, stool, and urine.

Multiple studies have measured the amount of toxins removed from the body and collected in the sweat. These include studies that investigated the removal of heavy metals such as mercury through the infrared sauna.[1] In addition to heavy metals, many other environmental chemicals such as pesticides and PCBs can be eliminated by sauna therapy.[2-4] Since we do not have any other good way to eliminate many of the toxins in our environment, sauna therapy is a good method that can be done very safely before pregnancy.

In addition to its effects on detoxification, the infrared sauna has other health benefits for people with chronic pain, arthritis, fatigue, and even heart disease.[5] It appears to decrease oxidative stress and inflammation, which may be part of the reason it improves health.[6]

For prepregnant women, ideal use would be three times a week for three to six months duration. Anyone with a chronic illness or known toxic exposure should do a longer protocol. I recommend starting slowly at five minutes a day and work up to 30 minutes. If tired or sick the following day, I recommend reducing the time spent in the sauna. The temperature at initial sauna sessions should be around 100 degrees. Later sessions should be at 130 degrees. It is important to not become dehydrated and to have enough electrolytes (sodium and potassium) along with minerals such as calcium and magnesium.

Since sauna is heating the body, it is important not to do sauna therapy during pregnancy for the same reasons that hot tub therapy is not recommended.

Detoxification Protocols

In the prior chapter, I discussed formulas to strengthen detoxification. These combination formulas use enzymes, amino acids, vitamins, minerals, herbs such as chlorella, and glutathione needed to bind heavy metals and other toxins. Formulas with these ingredients are meant to be slow and safe heavy metal detoxifiers. They should be taken 1 to 2 doses a day for the length of the detoxification protocol. Depending on symptoms and history of illness, a period of three to six months should be adequate.

The herbs chlorella, which is a green algae, and cilantro work well to remove toxins when taken together. Again, they are taken on a daily basis with the goal to have a slow detoxification of heavy metals along with fat-soluble toxins such as dioxin.

Health care practitioners, trained in environmental medicine and heavy metal detoxification, will often use prescription medicines such as DMSA (dimercaptosuccinic acid), DMPS (2,3-dimercapto-pro-pane-sulfonate), or EDTA (ethylenediaminetetraccetic acid) to bind metals. These can be very effective but need to be used safely and under medical supervision.

Stopping Toxic Habits
Smoking

The dangers of smoking, from heart disease to cancer, are well known. Yet for women considering pregnancy, smoking poses additional risks to the mother and her child. Smoking increases the risk for miscarriages. It leads to smaller size infants with an increased risk of stillbirth, congenital defects, and early infant deaths. Smoking literally decreases blood circulation leading to lower oxygen concentrations in the infant. This decreased oxygen to the brain may be the reason why children who were exposed to smoke in utero have a slower ability to learn. Smoking leads to a higher rate of breathing problems in infants including recurrent colds, pneumonia, and asthma. Infants who are exposed to nicotine in utero may have an increased likelihood of smoking addiction when they become older.

Cigarette smoking contains numerous dangerous toxins, including neurotoxins.

Toxins in cigarettes

- Nicotine (an addictive chemical)
- Pesticides from growing tobacco
- Heavy metals: cadmium, arsenic, and lead
- Vinyl chloride
- Formaldehyde
- Solvents such as benzene, pyrene, and benzopyrene
- Carbon monoxide
- Radioactive compounds
- Nitrosamine compounds

Obviously the answer for smokers is to quit smoking, something easier said than done. It takes most smokers more than one try to quit and they often feel terrible in the process. Help is available and should be utilized. For the health of the mother and the baby, it is very important to quit several months beforehand and give the woman's body enough time to detoxify and recover.

After quitting smoking, a woman's detox program should include extra nutrients depleted by smoking such as vitamin C in high doses of at least 3 gms or (3000 mgs) a day, additional beta-carotene, vitamin A 5,000 IUs, zinc 30 mg, selenium 200 mcg, and vitamin E (form that includes all forms of vitamin E) 400-800 IUs. A source of glutathione is also important since smoking depletes this important anti-oxidant. Glutathione can be inhaled to help heal the lungs.

Alcohol and Other Recreational Drugs

It is important to stop all alcohol and recreational drugs before pregnancy. If a woman cannot do this, professional help is warranted. Exposure to alcohol during pregnancy causes Fetal Alcohol Syndrome with specific changes to facial features and lifelong learning and developmental delays including ADHD. There is no health benefit from alcohol or other recreational drugs.

Alcohol also depletes nutrients in the body and puts additional strain on the liver. Additional liver support such as milk thistle, glutathione and vitamin C is needed for anyone who consumes alcohol.

Prescription Medications

Women considering pregnancy should review each of their prescription medicines with their physician. Medications are coded for whether they are safe to use during pregnancy. Medicines that could overtly cause birth defects are highlighted. However, medicines listed as safe may still have deleterious health effects to a pregnant woman and her baby.

Many women take antidepressants and some are deemed safe during pregnancy. One recent study found that antidepressants induce autism-like gene expression in fish.[7] Another study raised concerns about the effects of antidepressants on the nervous systems of newborns.[8] Finally, a third study found that antidepressant use during the first trimester may increase the risk of autism.[9] However, there are also risks to the mother and her offspring from depression, so the decision to stop this medication needs to happen with the advice of a physician. It can take many months or up to a year to wean-off an antidepressant. Additional nutritional support is helpful, including additional B vitamins, amino acid precursors of neurotransmitters (such as forms of tryptophan and/or tyrosine), and herbs that can support mood such as St John's Wort. Stress reduction, sleep, good diet, and exercise are also important when reducing the use of antidepressants.

Summary

After learning about the health effects of the vast number of toxins in our environment, I hope it is evident that addressing the environment is an important part of preparing for pregnancy. Begin with education and avoidance. Equally important is strengthening the body's ability to eliminate toxins. This should be followed by a safe detoxification plan (again, only before pregnancy). For women and men with chronic health issues, working with an experienced health practitioner for a more comprehensive plan is highly recommended.

CHAPTER 14 REFERENCES

1. Lovejoy HB, Bell ZG, Vizena TR. Mercury exposure evaluations and their correlation with urine mercury excretion: 4. Elimination of mercury by sweating. *J Occup Med.* 1973. 15:5900-591. DH581.

2. Schnare DW, Ben M, Shields MG. Body burden reductions of PCB's, PBB's, and chlorinated pesticides in human subjects. *Ambio*, 1984. 13;5-6:378-80. DH582.

3. Roehm DC. Effects of a program of sauna baths and megavitamins on adipose DDE and PCB's and on clearing of symptoms of agent orange (Dioxin) toxicity. *Clin Res.* 1983. 31;2:243A. DH583.

4. Rea WJ, Pan Y, Fenyves EJ, et al. Reduction of chemicals sensitivity by means of heat depuration, physical therapy and nutritional supplementation in a controlled environment. *J Nutr Environ Med.* 1996. 7;2:141-48. DH584.

5. Crinnion WJ. Sauna as a valuable clinical tool for cardiovascular, autoimmune, toxicant- induced and other chronic health problems. *Altern Med Rev.* 2011 Sep;16(3):215-25. PMID 21951023. DH526.

6. Masuda A, Miyata M, Kihara T, Minagoe S, Tei C. Repeated sauna therapy reduces urinary 8-epi-prostaglandin F(2alpha). *Jpn Heart J.* 2004 Mar;45(2):297-303. DH585.

7. Thomas MA, Klaper RD. Psychoactive Pharmaceuticals Induce Fish Gene Expression Profiles Associated with Human Idiopathic Autism. *PLoS ONE.* 2012 Jun:7(6). DH527.

8. Nijenhuis CM, Horst PG, Berg LT, Wilffert B. Disturbed development of the enteric nervous system after in utero exposure of selective serotonin re-uptake inhibitors and tricyclic antidepressants. Part 1: Literature review. *Br J Clin Pharmacol.* 2012 Jan;73(1):16-26. DH528.

9. Croen LA, Grether JK, Yoshida CK, Odouli R, Hendrick V. Antidepressant use during pregnancy and childhood autism spectrum disorders. *Arch Gen Psychiatry.* 2011 Nov;68(11):1104-12. 21727247. DH388.

Part 3

Pregnancy and Delivery
Autism & ADHD Prevention

15

Special Diet and Supplement Considerations

A woman completely supports the physical development of her child from the moment of conception until the end of breast-feeding. The food she consumes, the medicines she takes, and the chemicals she is exposed to are shared with the child. During pregnancy, the mother and her baby are intertwined in a mother-baby health bond.

Increased Nutrient Needs

All the nutrients for the baby in utero must be supplied by the mother. This includes extra vitamins and minerals, along with extra calories, extra protein, and even extra fluids. The nutritional status of the mother before and during pregnancy directly influences the child's birth weight and overall health. The amount of extra calories needed depends on the trimester. The American Congress of Obstetricians and Gynecologists (ACOG) makes recommendations for additional caloric intake and weight gain. On average, a woman should eat an additional 300 calories per day. Recommended weight increase during pregnancy depends on a woman's body mass index. Underweight women should gain 35 pounds, normal weight women should gain 15 to 35 pounds and obese women should gain 11 to 20 pounds.[1]

Increased nutrient needs exist for protein and some specific nutrients that tend to run low in many women's diets. Most women eat about 45 grams of protein per day. An extra 30 grams of protein per day is recommended[2] starting from the second month of pregnancy. This extra 30 grams can be met by 3 ounces of meat, 2 cups of beans, or 3 cups of milk or yogurt. The protein should be a complete protein that contains all of the amino acids: either animal protein or a balanced combination of vegetable proteins. Meat protein is a good source of iron and zinc that are also needed during pregnancy.

Dietary fats, including cholesterol and essential fatty acids, are also important for pregnancy. This is not the time to consider a low fat diet. The brain is made up of approximately 60% fat. During the first trimester the structure of the nervous system is formed which requires fat. The fat needs of the baby continue to increase, especially during the third trimester when the largest transfer of DHA for the baby's brain takes place. It is essential for the infant's proper development for the mother to have adequate DHA in her diet from sources like fish oil. If there is not enough fat in the mother's diet, the DHA will preferentially be passed to the baby lowering the mother's DHA level. Lower DHA levels are also associated with postpartum depression.[3]

Pregnant women often have low levels of calcium, iron, zinc, and folic acid. The supplements and diet recommendations from Part 2 should help women to go into pregnancy with adequate levels of important vitamins and minerals.

Calcium

During pregnancy, calcium is needed for the baby's bones, teeth, and other tissues. Women need an extra 400 mg of calcium a day for a total of 1200 mg.[4] With 3 to 4 servings of dairy plus a prenatal vitamin (often 200 mg of calcium), most women will have adequate intake. If a woman does not consume dairy products, an additional 800 to 1000 mg a day should be supplemented.

Magnesium

Many pregnancy books neglect to mention that additional magnesium is needed to balance calcium intake. Magnesium in many women's diets is low. In fact, it is one of the most common mineral deficiencies in the U.S. An extra 350 mg of magnesium is needed daily.

Benefits of magnesium

- For bone health (when balanced with calcium)
- Decreases headaches and constipation (relaxes muscles)
- Promotes sleep (take before bed on an empty stomach)
- Decreases premature contractions
- Decreases elevated blood pressure in pregnancy (called *preeclampsia*)

Iron

Pregnancy requires extra iron. The iron in a quality prenatal vitamin is usually adequate. The woman's doctor will normally run a complete blood count test to screen for iron. However, the additional ferritin test will give an earlier indication of low iron levels. A good ferritin level is 50.

Zinc

Zinc is important for reproductive health and is especially important during the first trimester as the baby's neurologic system begins forming. In addition to the zinc in their prenatal vitamin, women should add an extra 15 mg of highly absorbable zinc such as zinc picolinate or zinc chelate.

Vitamin C

Vitamin C is important for collagen development that helps to form the structure of our tissues. Fruits and vegetables are good sources of vitamin C. A woman that takes a daily prenatal vitamin and consumes lots of fruits or vegetables is probably getting enough vitamin C, but most women need to take an extra 500 to 1000 mg since it is safe and beneficial.

Folinic acid and B vitamins

Pregnant women need to take extra amounts of some vitamins, including folic acid in the active form of methylfolate or folinic acid. This should be taken with the active form of vitamin B12 or methylcobalamin. Most prenatal vitamins do not have these forms so individual supplements may be needed. A B-complex vitamin with the active forms or coenzyme forms will work well. The B vitamins are water-soluble so the extra B vitamins are safe. It is crucial to have these vitamins in the first trimester when the nervous system is being formed. These B vitamins, especially folinic acid and B12, are needed to prevent neural tube defects. Vitamin B6 appears to be helpful as well. These B vitamins, which are important for the biochemical process of methylation, appear also to help prevent Down syndrome.[5]

Caution: All supplements should be reviewed and approved by a woman's physician before use.

Summary of recommended supplements during pregnancy:

- Prenatal vitamin
- High DHA fish oil: 1000 mg of fish oil (750 mg from DHA and 250 mg from EPA)
- Probiotics: combination of lactobacillus and acidophilus
- Vitamin D: 1000 IUs (more may be needed depending on blood levels)
- Methylfolate: 800 mcg (in prenatal vitamin or additional B-complex vitamin)
- Methyl B12: 200 mcg (in prenatal vitamin or additional B-complex vitamin)
- Calcium: 800 mg (if no dairy intake)
- Magnesium: 350 mg total (100 mg is often in prenatal vitamin)

Supplements during prepregnancy and pregnancy

It is important to recognize that there are some key differences in the amounts and forms of supplements between the preconception period and pregnancy. One of the main differences concerns the amounts of the fat-soluble vitamins: vitamin A (in cod liver oil) and vitamin

D. High doses of vitamin A during pregnancy can cause birth defects, especially if ingested during the first trimester.[6] Therefore, a women should not take more than 1 teaspoon of cod liver oil per day. From research studies it appears that high doses of vitamin D are safe and probably needed during pregnancy.[7] But since vitamin D is a fat-soluble vitamin, if a woman does not know what her blood vitamin D level is, she can take 1,000 IUs in addition to the amount in the prenatal vitamin. The amounts of methylfolate and B12 are also lower. The goal before pregnancy is to take higher doses to build up nutrient stores. Then during pregnancy, a woman is safely supplementing for a healthy pregnancy in amounts that are adequate but not too high.

Risks of Maternal Malnutrition

If a mother is malnourished with insufficient calories and nutrients she will not have the needed increase in blood volume to support proper placental growth. A decrease in placental growth is associated with lower birth weight and its resulting medical complications.[8]

Deficits in specific nutrients can also lead to complications in pregnancy, several of which can increase the risk of preterm delivery. A lack of vitamins that support methylation (B6, B12, folinic acid, and choline) is associated with increased risk of neural tube defects.[9,10] Decreased calcium and magnesium intakes are associated with *preeclampsia*,[11,12] which is elevated blood pressure in pregnancy that leads to early delivery and small infants. Preeclampsia can also cause severe health consequences to the mother (such as seizures) if not treated early.

Avoiding Seafood

Seafood is a good source of protein and the essential fatty acids (both DHA and EPA). Unfortunately, many of our lakes, rivers, and oceans are contaminated with mercury. Mercury concentrates higher up the food chain so mercury in the smaller fish passes to the bigger fish when they are eaten. Currently the medical community endorses fish consumption by pregnant women albeit with limits to avoid excessive mercury. The problem with this approach is that mercury, even in small amounts, is very neurotoxic to a developing fetus. Mercury causes neurologic development problems similar to the symptoms of autism.[13] Therefore, as a precaution, I do not recommend that pregnant women eat any fish—especially during the first trimester when the nervous system is first being formed.

If a woman does not eat fish during pregnancy, she can make up the nutrients in other ways. There are multiple safe sources of protein available and fish oil capsules that have been tested for mercury and for PCBs. With safe alternatives available, it does not make sense to me to risk the baby's health with mercury exposure that can easily be controlled by diet.

If a pregnant woman chooses to eat fish (hopefully not during the first trimester), she should choose fish low in mercury. The National Resource Defense Council has a guide to mercury levels in various fish species at www.nrdc.org/mercury. The highest levels of mercury are found in king mackerel, marlin, orange roughy, shark, swordfish, tilefish, and tuna. These fish are not recommended for pregnant women or young children.

Seafood has other concerns in addition to mercury. While salmon is one of the least mercury-containing fish, much of the salmon supply today is grown in farms that have other risks. Farmed salmon have less omega-3 fats because they are not eating algae in the ocean to incorporate these oils. The water in the fish farms is usually not as clean as in the wild and can be contaminated with toxic chemicals such as PCBs that cause health problems. Shellfish can contain arsenic that is another heavy metal that can negatively affect the nervous system and should be avoided.

Alcohol

We know that there is nothing nutritional in alcohol. We also know that alcohol can negatively affect a child's growth and cause serious long-term developmental consequences in infants. Yet as many as 12 percent of women drink some alcohol during pregnancy.[14] About half of infants born to women who are alcoholics will have fetal alcohol syndrome, which is a permanent lifelong developmental delay. Thus, heavy alcohol use will harm the new baby. Various studies have shown that light drinking may be safe during pregnancy, however as a precautionary measure I recommend pregnant women consume no alcohol at all.

Foods to avoid

Similar to the foods to avoid before pregnancy listed in Chapter 5, here is a list of foods to avoid during pregnancy:

- Genetically Modified foods (GMs)
- Artificial sweeteners (sucralose with trademark Splenda and Aspartame)
- Foods with MSG
- High fructose corn syrup
- Trans fats
- Food dyes
- Food preservatives (benzoic acid, calcium and potassium benzoate, BHA, BHT, or nitrites)
- High-mercury foods, including seafood
- Alcohol

Foods to Minimize

Caffeine

Pregnant women are advised to limit their intake of caffeine. As a stimulant, it increases heart rate and causes blood vessels to constrict. Obviously during pregnancy constriction of blood vessels to the baby is not good. High use of caffeine early in pregnancy is correlated with increased rates of miscarriages.[15] Most physicians advise pregnant women to limit caffeine intake to about 1 cup a day. Since tea, especially green tea, has less caffeine switching from coffee to green tea is a good choice. Even two cups of green tea has less caffeine than one cup of coffee. Green tea also has many anti-oxidants so it is both a safer and healthier choice.

Caffeine can also stress adrenal hormones. Caffeine triggers a release of fight or flight hormones that can lead to adrenal fatigue. A pregnant woman's adrenals are already working hard and further depleting the adrenals will lead to increased fatigue and immune weakness.

A recent study also found that caffeine may affect the neurotransmitter serotonin,[16] which is needed for regulation of mood, appetite, and sleep. It also helps memory and learning.

There are also concerns about using caffeine during the last part of pregnancy. The fetus and newborn infant appear to lack the enzymes necessary to demethylate or metabolize caffeine. Therefore, a newborn detoxifying from caffeine will be more irritable and fussy.

Sugar

In pregnancy, women can develop *gestational diabetes*. This is elevated blood sugar or diabetes that happens for the first time in pregnancy. Women are screened for this disorder during the second trimester. Controlling sugar and simple carbohydrate intake is important for preventing the subsequent spikes in insulin associated with gestational diabetes. When the insulin levels are elevated frequently, this can lead to insulin resistance and gestational diabetes. Gestational diabetes ends when the baby is born but sets-up women for developing type 2 or insulin resistance diabetes as they get older. Gestational diabetes during pregnancy is correlated with many pregnancy and newborn complications.[17] These infants tend to be large which leads to pregnancy and delivery complications. Their metabolism has a problem regulating blood sugar. They can have developmental delays and often have problems feeding. And, importantly, researchers have correlated an increased risk of autism with mothers who had gestational diabetes.[18]

Ways to avoid high blood sugar and insulin problems

- Smaller, frequent meals with protein and good fats
- Decreased simple carbohydrates like white bread and pasta
- Decreased sugars (also helps with digestion and avoiding yeast infections)
- Avoid high fructose sugars and high sugar foods like refined fruit juices and soda

Caution Labeling: Pregnancy Categories

Medicines and herbs are categorized for safety during pregnancy and breastfeeding (see Table 15.1). For pregnancy, they are given the categories: A, B, C, D, and X. These categories are listed for prescriptions so any medicine or herb or supplement taken needs to be checked for its categorization as described below. Any medicine or herb in category A is safe for all pregnant women. Categories B and C mean we really do not know if they are safe. Any product in these categories needs to be discussed between the pregnant woman and her health care provider to look at the risk/benefit ratio. The last two categories D and X should not be taken.

Table 15.1 - Caution Labeling of Products During Pregnancy

Label	Warning
A	*Adequate studies in pregnant women have not demonstrated a risk to the fetus in the first trimester of pregnancy, and there is no evidence of risk in later trimesters.*
B	*Animal studies have not demonstrated a risk to the fetus, but there are no adequate studies in pregnant women or animal studies that have shown an adverse effect but adequate studies in pregnant women have not shown a risk to the fetus.*
C	*Animal studies have shown an adverse effect on the fetus but there are no adequate human studies (note the difference between human and animal studies).*
D	*There is evidence of human fetal risk but the potential benefits for the pregnant women may be acceptable despite the risks.*
X	*Studies in animals or humans demonstrate clear evidence of fetal risk that outweigh the possible benefit in a pregnant woman.*

Over the Counter Medicines

If possible, a pregnant woman should avoid over-the-counter medicines unless directed by a doctor. Medicines require the body to detoxify. One medicine that is supposedly safe for pregnant women is Tylenol or acetaminophen. I am concerned with Tylenol because it can be very harmful to the liver at doses just above safe levels. With a pregnant mother, we need to be extra careful. Tylenol is metabolized by the liver and depletes the largest anti-oxidant in the body: glutathione. Depleting glutathione weakens the body by decreasing its ability to detoxify. However, since both ibuprofen and aspirin can increase risk of bleeding, neither of them is recommended in pregnancy, which has led to the recommendation of Tylenol as the only safe pain reliever.

Prescription Medicines

Any woman on prescription medicines needs to work with their doctor to make sure that each medicine is essential. It should be the safest type of medicine and the lowest effective dose.

Examples of common medicines and pregnancy label category

- Acetaminophen (Tylenol™): B
- Ibuprofen (Advil™): B/D
- Aspirin: C/D
- Ranitidine (Zantac™) acid blocker: B
- Amoxicillin (antibiotic): B
- Fluoxetine (Prozac™) for depression: C
- Sertraline (Zoloft™) for depression: C

High-Dose Supplements

Caution should be taken when ingesting any supplement, especially supplements in high doses. Anytime additional amounts of one nutrient are added, the possibility exists that it may affect or imbalance another nutrient in the body. A woman should always check with her doctor before taking supplements.

Herbs

The reason that many herbs are beneficial for our health is because they have chemical constituents that support our bodies. In fact, many prescription medicines are originally from herbs. Therefore any herb taken in pregnancy must be shown to be safe in pregnancy—again, a woman should check first with her doctor.

Some cultures have used specific herbs, often in tea form, for centuries and modern medicine considers them safe for pregnant women. The main ingredient in many pregnancy teas is the leaf from the herb red raspberry. Red raspberry leaf tea is known for strengthening the uterus. Chamomile tea is calming and safe and can be helpful for upset stomachs.

Treatments for Morning Sickness

Morning sickness can last all day and is common in the first trimester. Medical research shows that the herb ginger is safe and effective for morning sickness.[19] It can be taken in capsules or as a tea. The following are also safe and effective treatments for morning sickness:

- Raspberry leaf tea
- Peppermint tea
- Vitamin B6: 25 to 50 mg per day, reduce fatty foods, increase carbohydrates and have small frequent meals
- Eating a few dry crackers upon waking in the morning
- Some women may get relief from acupuncture or acupressure by a trained professional

Luckily for most women after the first trimester ends, the nausea passes.

Summary

Pregnancy is a unique time when everything a mother consumes can affect her growing infant, either positively or negatively. Since the unborn child is so small and vulnerable the utmost care needs to be taken to protect the child. All the crucial nutrients to grow a healthy nervous system need to be provided in adequate amounts. Pregnancy is the time to maintain proper nutrition and benefit from the stores created before pregnancy in order to maximize the future health of the child and avoid autism and ADHD.

CHAPTER 15 REFERENCES

1. American Congress of Obstetricians and Gynecologists. Nutrition During Pregnancy Fact Sheet. Accessed 1/13/13. DH529.

2. Sardesai V. National Research Council. *Introduction to Clinical Nutrition*. 2012: 12.2.3.2. 286. DH530

3. Ibid.

4. Ibid.

5. Zampieri BL, Biselli JM, Goloni-Bertollo EM, Vannucchi H, Carvalho VM, Cordeiro JA, Pavarino EC. Maternal risk for Down syndrome is modulated by genes involved in folate metabolism. *Dis Markers*. 2012;32(2):73-81. DH533.

6. Rothman KJ, Moore LL, Singer MR, Nguyen US, Mannino S, Milunsky A. Teratogenicity of high vitamin A intake. *N Engl J Med*. 1995 Nov 23;333(21):1369-73. DH534.

7. Hollis BW, Wagner CL. Vitamin D requirements during lactation: high-dose maternal supplementation as therapy to prevent hypovitaminosis D for both the mother and the nursing infant. *Am J Clin Nutr*. 2004 Dec:80(6 Suppl):1752S-1758S. DH316.

8. Mathews F, Youngman L, Neil A. Maternal circulating nutrient concentrations in pregnancy: implications for birth and placental weights of term infants. *Am J Clin Nutr*. 2004 Jan;79(1):103-10. DH535.

9. Schorah CJ, Smithells RW. Primary prevention of neural tube defects with folic acid. *BMJ*. 1993;306(6885):1123-1124. DH19.

10. Thompson MD, Cole DE, Ray JG. Vitamin B-12 and neural tube defects: the Canadian experience. *Am J Clin Nutr*. 2009;89(2):697S-701S. DH20.

11. Romero-Arauz JF, Morales-Borrego E, García-Espinosa M, Peralta-Pedrero ML. Clinical guideline. Preeclampsia-eclampsia. *Rev Med Inst Mex Seguro Soc*. 2012 Sep-Oct;50(5):569-79. DH536.

12. Patrelli TS, Dall'asta A, Gizzo S, Pedrazzi G, Piantelli G, Jasonni VM, Modena AB. Calcium supplementation and prevention of preeclampsia: a meta-analysis. *J Matern Fetal Neonatal Med*. 2012 Dec;25(12):2570-4. DH537.

13. Mutter J, Naumann J, Schneider R, Walach H, Haley B. Mercury and autism: accelerating evidence? *Neuro Endocrinol Lett*. 2005:26(5):436-446. DH301.

14. Pruett D, Waterman EH, Caughey AB. Fetal alcohol exposure: consequences, diagnosis, and treatment. *Obstet Gynecol Surv.*. 2013 Jan;68(1):62-9.DH538.

15. Greenwood DC, Alwan N, Boylan S, Cade JE, Charvill J, Chipps KC, Cooke MS, Dolby VA, Hay AW, Kassam S, Kirk SF, Konje JC, Potdar N, Shires S, Simpson N, Taub N, Thomas JD, Walker J, White KL, Wild CP. Caffeine intake during pregnancy, late miscarriage and stillbirth. *Eur J Epidemiol.* 2010 Apr;25(4):275-80. DH539.

16. Li XD, He RR, Qin Y, Tsoi B, Li YF, Ma ZL, Yang X, Kurihara H. Caffeine interferes embryonic development through over-stimulating serotonergic system in chicken embryo. *Food Chem Toxicol.* 2012 Jun;50(6):1848-53. DH619.

17. Negrato CA, Mattar R, Gomes MB. Adverse pregnancy outcomes in women with diabetes. *Diabetol Metab Syndr.* 2012 Sep 11;4(1):41. DH540.

18. Krakowiak P, Walker CK, Bremer AA, Baker AS, Ozonoff S, Hansen RL, Hertz-Picciotto I. Maternal metabolic conditions and risk for autism and other neurodevelopmental disorders. *Pediatrics.* 2012 May;129(5):e1121-8. DH541.

19. Ding M, Leach M, Bradley H. The effectiveness and safety of ginger for pregnancy-induced nausea and vomiting: A systematic review. *Women Birth.* 2012 Aug 27. DH542.

16

Environment, Toxins, and Vaccines

Apregnant woman needs to be vigilant to protect herself and her baby from potential environmental harm. Everything a pregnant woman eats, drinks, touches, or breathes should be as safe as possible. Avoidance of toxins, especially during the first trimester is very important. If in doubt, a woman should go without!

Since is not safe to detoxify during pregnancy, toxin avoidance is the best strategy. The Part 2 toxin chapters described the most important chemicals to avoid, including chemicals from food, water, cosmetics, and cleaners. Other sources are work-related, outdoor air pollutants and lawn pesticides.

During pregnancy, there are some other potential toxin exposures to consider.

Dental-Related Exposures

If a woman has metal dental amalgams in her mouth, having a general dental cleaning could potentially increase mercury exposure. Hopefully women will not go into pregnancy with mercury containing amalgams, but if it happens, extreme care needs to be taken during dental appointments. This is definitely not the time for getting amalgam fillings removed or replaced.

X-Rays

Another potential dental concern is the use of dental x-rays. It is important to avoid all non-critical exposure to radiation. Most routine dental x-rays can wait until the pregnancy is over. The radiation risk is greatest for a fetus from 2 to 15 weeks post-conception.[1] Studies of pregnant women indicate that excess radiation can terminate pregnancy, restrict fetal growth and harm neurologic development. Doses above the dose of 100 mGy (10 rad) may cause a decrease in their child's IQ.[2] Radiation may also increase the risk of cancer in the child. When x-rays are deemed critical to the health of the mother, then all precautions need to be taken to protect the fetus.

Electromagnetic Fields (EMFs)

Flowing electrical current in devices generate electromagnetic fields. Since research has raised concerns regarding EMFs harming fertility and causing health problems, it makes sense that precautions should be taken during pregnancy. From a review of the literature, it appears that we really do not know yet the impact of EMFs on pregnancy and future child health.

Since we do not know the risks, for assuring the health of the baby it makes sense to decrease exposure as much as possible. If, in the future, EMFs are found to be low risk, a woman may be merely inconvenienced for 9 months. If however, EMFs are found to be harmful to the baby, then she would have avoided a negative health impact on her baby.

One of the most prevalent sources of EMFs is cell phones. A woman should keep her cell phone off of her body. The whole idea of a cell phone being carried next to a developing fetus is very frightening. A safe headset can be worn when a cell phone needs to be used. The phone should be turned off as much as possible. Women should avoid sleeping next to a cell phone or even an electrical alarm clock. There is a difference in how much a specific type of cell phone emits EMFs. Each cell phone should be checked and lower radiation phones should be used. Electrical appliances such as a computer should be kept off the lap. One study found that laptop computers used by pregnant women generate electrical currents in the fetus.[3] The computer wireless network should be turned off at night. Women should even consider replacing their wireless house phones with corded phones.

An additional source of EMFs is proximity to utility electric power lines. Again, research has not conclusively determined health risks from high power transmission lines. But as a precaution, I recommend women not live near them during pregnancy if at all possible.

I realize that some people may question the need for these actions, but protection from potential harm (even harm we do not fully understand) may turn out to be very important for the health of the child.

Vaccines
Influenza vaccine

There are several vaccines that are recommended for pregnant women. The most common one is the flu or influenza. Flu vaccination is given because pregnant woman and their infants are considered high risk for problems if they contact the flu.

One of the primary concerns with the flu vaccine is that many manufacturers still include the mercury preservative thimerosal. Since we know that mercury is a neurotoxin and the fetus is developing a nervous system, exposing the infant to a known dose of mercury does not make any sense. Preservative-free flu shots are available. There are other ingredients in the influenza vaccine, such as formaldehyde, that may harm the fetus.

One of the primary concerns with the flu shot was raised in 2011, by a study[4] published in the journal *Vaccine*. The study showed that the influenza vaccine caused measurable amounts of inflammatory response in the mother's body. While limited inflammatory response from a vaccine is normal (this is how immunity is created) the inflammation identified in this study present real concerns for a pregnant woman. What are the effects from the increased inflammatory markers on the health of a developing baby in utero? We do know that multiple diseases contain an inflammatory component, including pregnancy complications such as preterm birth and preeclampsia. We also know that autism is a disease with a large inflammatory component and that one of our ways toward prevention of autism is to decrease inflammation and inflammatory markers.

In 2012, a research study was released showing that a woman who had influenza during pregnancy had a twofold increase chance of having a child with autism.[5] Why this correlation exists is unclear. Some practitioners will use this as evidence that women should get the influenza vaccine during pregnancy. The problem with this is that when a person gets an influenza vaccine, their body is exposed to parts of the virus in order to produce an immune and inflammatory response. With this concept in mind, we may actually be causing an immune response that will increase the risk of autism. Another reason that influenza in pregnancy may be associated with autism could be the increased use of Tylenol in women who develop influenza. We know there are concerns with Tylenol's effect on liver function and glutathione depletion.

Instead of only relying on the influenza vaccination, a woman should strengthen her immune system to avoid getting influenza. Research does show that adequate levels of vitamin D helps to prevent influenza.[6] Elderberry syrup has been shown to be safe and effective for influenza prevention and treatment.[7]

Each woman needs to take into account her individual situation and discuss with her doctor the risks and benefits of the influenza vaccine.

Rhogam

Rhogam or Rho(D) immune globulin is given only to women who have a negative blood type such as A-, B-, AB-, or O-. This is given to protect the mother from having an antibody response to her fetus if the fetus's blood type is positive. The antibodies formed by a mother with a negative blood type can potentially lead to bleeding or stillbirth in her newborn.

Before 2001, Rhogam contained the mercury preservative thimerosal. Research from infants born to women who had Rhogam inoculation with thimerosal showed mixed results for any connection with autism. The interesting fact is that the researchers who did find positive correlation between the Rhogam shot with thimerosal are those who treat children with autism and had much greater knowledge of their issues. At this point no other issues have been raised and Rhogam can be life-saving, so if a woman has a negative blood type there is often good justification that she receives this vaccine when recommended by her physician. It is important to check to make sure it is preservative-free.

Tdap (Tetanus, Diphtheria and Pertussis)

In 2011, the CDC recommended that pregnant women that have never received the Tdap vaccine be inoculated against the diseases diphtheria, tetanus, and pertussis. *Tetanus* is prolonged contraction of skeletal muscular fibers (like lockjaw). Tetanus has largely been eradicated in developed countries. *Diphtheria* is an upper respiratory illness that has almost been completely eradicated in the U.S. *Pertussis*, which is whooping cough in a newborn infant, can be very serious.

Concerns have been raised that giving a pregnant woman this vaccine may have a negative impact on the infant's immunity to later vaccines. Clinical trials are ongoing to address this concern. Similar issues need to be addressed with the use of this vaccine as with the use of the influenza vaccine. What is the impact of vaccine additives such as formaldehyde on a developing fetus? All vaccines create an inflammatory response and how does this affect the long-term health of the infant and the risk of autism? Again, women should consult with their doctors on this vaccine.

MMR (Measles, Mumps and Rubella)

This combined vaccine protects against the respiratory infection *measles*, a virus that produces swelling called *mumps* and the rash-producing virus *rubella* (also called *German measles*).

The CDC does not recommend the MMR vaccine for pregnant women. It is also recommended that women not become pregnant for 28 days after the vaccine.

A pregnant woman will be screened to see if she has been exposed to rubella. This is often done in early pregnancy since exposure to rubella during pregnancy can lead to birth defects. If a woman has never been exposed to rubella, obstetricians will often recommend vaccination with the MMR vaccine after pregnancy and during nursing. However, as will be described in Chapter 21, there are numerous concerns with this practice.

Summary

Pregnancy is an important time to avoid any potential toxin exposure. This includes any foreign substance if its safety is not proven. The future mother should avoid x-rays unless medically necessary. EMFs are a major concern because the amount of exposure has increased so rapidly that it is unavoidable but we have no idea if any amount is safe to an unborn child.

By definition, vaccines cause an inflammatory response in the mother. How this inflammatory response affects the immune system of the growing child is largely unknown. We have evidence that a vaccinated pregnant mother passes autoantibodies or immune proteins to their developing fetus—is there a relation to autism? Vaccines prevent diseases but carry risks, especially during the vulnerable time of pregnancy. Women should consult with trained medical professionals for the best decisions for them and their children.

1. Williams PM, Fletcher S. Health effects of prenatal radiation exposure. *Am Fam Physician.* 2010 Sep 1;82(5):488-93. DH544.

2. Timins JK. Radiation during pregnancy. *N J Med.* 2001 Jun;98(6):29-33. DH545.

3. Bellieni CV, Pinto I, Bogi A, Zoppetti N, Andreuccetti D, Buonocore G. Exposure to electromagnetic fields from laptop use of "laptop" computers. *Arch Environ Occup Health.* 2012;67(1):31-6. DH546.

4. Christian LM, Iams JD, Porter K, Glaser R. Inflammatory responses to trivalent influenza virus vaccine among pregnant women. *Vaccine.* 2011 Nov 8;29(48):8982-7. DH445.

5. Sumaya CV, Gibbs RS. Immunization of pregnant women with influenza A/New Jersey/76 virus vaccine: reactogenicity and immunogenicity in mother and infant. *J Infect Dis.* 1979 Aug;140(2):141-6. DH547.

6. Cannell JJ, Vieth R, Umhau JC, Holick MF, Grant WB, Madronich S, Garland CF, Giovannucci E. Epidemic influenza and vitamin D. *Epidemiol Infect.* 2006 Dec;134(6):1129-40. DH615.

7. Yates L, Pierce M, Stephens S, Mill AC, Spark P, Kurinczuk JJ, Valappil M, Brocklehurst P, Thomas SH, Knight M. Influenza A/H1N1v in pregnancy: an investigation of the characteristics and management of affected women and the relationship to pregnancy outcomes for mother and infant. *Health Technol Assess.* 2010 Jul;14(34):109-82. DH548.

17

Delivery

All women wish for a peaceful, normal delivery without intervention and complications. Women who are healthy going into pregnancy and are able to maintain this health throughout pregnancy have the best chance of having their delivery go smoothly. Yet complications can occur for any woman. Being prepared for potential problems is important in order to minimize the possible health risks to both mother and infant. This chapter discusses interventions commonly used to assist delivery along with standard procedures after the birth of the infant. Women need to discuss these issues with their health care practitioner before delivery.

Perinatal Risk Factors Associated with Autism

At least 10 published studies[1-10] in the past 10 years have examined perinatal (around the time of birth) risk factors for the development of autism. Risk factors identified are not always consistent across these studies.

Perinatal risk factors associated with autism

- Labor less than 1 hour
- Labor induction with Pitocin
- C-section delivery
- Abnormal presentation at birth
- Fetal distress
- Umbilical cord around the neck
- Increased number of delivery complications
- Abnormal gestational age (born too early or too late)
- Multiple births (twins or triplets)
- Birth injury or trauma
- Severe maternal bleeding at delivery
- Meconium aspiration (infant swallows contaminated amniotic fluid)
- Congenital malformations
- Low Apgar scores (low scores on appearance, pulse, grimaced facial expression, activity and respiration)
- Neonatal anemia (low iron)
- ABO blood type/RH incompatibility (problem between infant and mother's blood types leading to an immune reaction causing jaundice)
- Hyperbilirubinemia (jaundice in a newborn)
- Feeding difficulties
- Small for gestational age (small size for age of infant)

The more perinatal risk factors present, the higher the incidence of autism. However, one single factor appears not to be decisive. For example, a child born before 40 weeks (the last week of pregnancy) by C-section, after failed induction with Pitocin, who shows signs of fetal distress and low Apgar scores after birth, would have a higher risk of autism than a child born by C-section with no other problems.

Many of the above perinatal risk factors could result in decreased oxygen to the infant. Low oxygen has the potential to injure an infant's brain and lead to developmental delays.

It should be noted that some birth complications are caused by earlier problems in utero—not the birth process itself.

Again, individual perinatal risk factors probably do not greatly increase the risk of autism. But it is clear to me from attending many births and from my pediatric practice that children with autism usually have experienced many of the above risk factors. Therefore, it is extremely important to avoid any controllable risk factors, including the risk factors during birth.

Birthing Position

During a traditional hospital birth, women lay on their backs during labor. This is the easiest position for a doctor to deliver the baby and monitor the labor with electronic fetal monitors. Women in labor often find this position more painful as it restricts normal movement. This position can slow labor and lead to an increased risk of assisted deliveries and birth complications. More pain also leads to an increased use of pain medicines, which increase numbers of assisted deliveries including C-sections. A more natural position for birthing is squatting or being supported sitting up.

Medicine Use During Delivery

There are three types of medicines used routinely at delivery. These are Pitocin (which is used to increase contractions), anesthesia for pain control, and antibiotics to prevent or treat infections.

Pitocin birth induction

Pitocin is a synthetic form of the natural hormone oxytocin and is used to start or increase contractions. Pitocin is made from the pituitary gland of cattle. Two preservatives are added to stabilize the formula: acetic acid and chloretone. Of concern is that the natural hormone oxytocin, which is produced during labor, is disrupted by Pitocin. Pitocin blocks the production of natural oxytocin needed for human bonding and social interaction.

There is also a correlation between Pitocin use during delivery and an increased risk of autism.[11] Pitocin causes a decrease in the receptors in the developing brain so less oxytocin can bind. This decreases oxytocin's positive effect on the developing nervous system. Researchers have also found different genetic types of oxytocin receptors on cells (genetic polymorphisms). There may be some people with a genetic vulnerability to have increased problems from Pitocin. One research study found a strong predictive relationship between Pitocin use and subsequent ADHD.[12] Treatment with oxytocin is helpful for increasing social interactions in some children with autism, which is consistent with lack of oxytocin (from use of Pitocin) being a causal factor in the development of autism. The last twenty years have seen an increase use in Pitocin, which is also the same time period that has seen an increase in autism rates.

Pitocin speeds up labor by increasing the intensity and frequency of uterine contractions. These strong contractions can be very painful which leads to an increase in use of pain medicines or anesthesia. Some believe it also increases the risk of fetal distress and therefore the use of assisted deliveries.

Mothers should discuss use of Pitocin and their concerns with their doctor in advance of delivery.

Assisted Deliveries

If there are concerns about the mother or the infant during labor, the delivery can be expedited through mechanical means (vaginal) or via C-section (Caesarian section).

Mechanical means pull the infant and include the use forceps and vacuum. A C-section is when an incision is made across a woman's lower abdomen and then through the uterus. The baby is pulled out directly from the uterus.

Forceps and vacuum deliveries

Forceps have paddles that attach to each side of the baby's head in the vaginal canal. During a vacuum assist, suction is applied to the crown of the baby's head.

The primary concern with either of these deliveries is that the head and therefore the neck and the spinal cord of the newborn are physically pulled. This pulling force can potentially cause trauma to the nervous system. It often causes bruises and swelling on the newborn's scalp that can take several weeks to resolve.

C-section delivery

A C-section is often performed in response to problems during delivery. It can also be planned ahead of time if a woman already had one C-section or if the baby is in the wrong position for delivery, e.g. breech position. A C-section surgery includes the use of anesthesia. More women today are electing to have the baby born by C-section—a concerning trend given the positive health benefits of the vaginal delivery and several concerns about C-sections.

During a vaginal delivery hormones are released in the mother that spur lactation for breastfeeding and promote bonding with the baby. During a C-section, this hormone release does not occur. We still need to better understand the health effects of this lack of hormone release during C-sections.

Infants going through the vaginal canal obtain good (probiotic) bacteria from their mothers.[13,14,15] Infants from C-section births do not get that good bacteria and are more prone to digestive problems. As part of labor, they are also supposed to have the amniotic fluid literally squeezed from their lungs. Since this does not happen during C-sections, these infants tend to have more breathing problems with a subsequent increase in admissions to neonatal intensive care nurseries. If they are admitted for intensive care, multiple invasive procedures such as intravenous (IV) fluids and antibiotics are often administered. C-section deliveries, if scheduled ahead of time, are usually scheduled for 1 week before term (39 weeks instead of 40). Just this 1 week can increase the risk of learning disabilities such as autism and dyslexia.[16] With this knowledge, it is important to wait the full 40 weeks before having a C-section delivery, unless complications necessitate otherwise.

During a C-section, there is risk of infection and antibiotics are often used, which can comprise the good gut flora in the mother. The surgery necessarily cuts through the mother's abdominal muscles, and I speak from personal experience that recovery is slow and painful.

For these reasons, I believe for the best health outcome for both the mother and her child a vaginal birth should be allowed to proceed, unless a C-section is medically necessary.

Treatment after Assisted Deliveries (C-section, Forceps and Vacuum)

Assisted deliveries are sometimes unavoidable, so it is important to know what can be done to lessen the impact on the infant. Since the good bacteria vital for good immunity and digestion are not obtained through a C-section birth, the infant should be supplemented with probiotics. Infants may also receive good bacteria for their digestive and immune systems through nursing.

A certified craniosacral therapist or an osteopath trained to work with young children can gently adjust an infant soon after birth after an assisted delivery. This may prevent neurologic problems from developing. It would be good for infants from a vaginal delivery to also receive this treatment since sometimes it is not known from a routine vaginal delivery if there has been any disruption of the nervous system. It is my experience that infants have better sleep, are calmer, and even have less gastroesophageal reflux after these adjustments.

Anesthesia

Anesthesia is used to control pain during delivery. It is always used with a C-section surgery, but often used in other deliveries as well. The most common type of anesthesia is called *epidural* anesthesia where the medicine is injected into the epidural space in the lower back below the spinal cord. Anesthesia needs to be metabolized by the detoxification system in the mother, and depending on when the anesthesia is started, also by the infant. After a delivery with anesthesia, some infants are sleepier and take more time to begin nursing.[17] The long-term health effects of anesthesia on infants are unknown. Anesthesia has not yet been identified as an individual risk factor for autism development, although it often coexists with other risk factors such as assisted deliveries. Anesthesia can slow down labor and can increase the likelihood of needing assisted delivery including C-sections. It is best if anesthesia can be avoided. If it needs to be used, then using the lowest dose for the shortest amount of time is a good strategy for the health of the mother and infant.

An option for pain relief is the use of hydrotherapy or warm water baths. Some birthing centers offer this therapy and it can help avoid anesthesia and other birth complications such as assisted deliveries.

Antibiotics

Antibiotics, usually in the IV form, are routinely used when there is a risk of infection during delivery. Some doctors use them for all C-sections. Women are routinely checked for the bacteria Group B strep toward the end of pregnancy. If they are positive for the bacteria, the doctors will often give IV antibiotics during or just before delivery. Group B strep can cause serious infections in a newborn infant if they obtain the strep bacteria during delivery. The problem with the use of antibiotics is that it kills much of the good bacteria in the intestines of the mother. The infant then does not get the good bacteria either from delivery or during nursing. Antibiotics can be life saving for infants and mothers, so their use is sometimes unavoidable. However, routine use should be curtailed when the risks of infection are minimal in order to maintain the mother's immune system and for a good start of the baby's immune system.

If antibiotics are used, both the mother and baby should be supplemented with higher doses of probiotics after delivery. Should the mother or infant present with digestive symptoms following delivery, additional probiotics may be needed.

Post-Delivery Procedures

Following the delivery, there are several standard practices done for the newborn infant including cutting the umbilical cord, placing antibiotic drops in the infant's eyes, and giving them a vitamin K injection.

Timing of cord clamping

For many years, standard practice for obstetricians was to cut the umbilical cord quickly after the birth of the baby, usually within 1 minute after birth. It was thought that too much blood going to the infant would be harmful. Recently it has been discovered that a longer time to clamp the cord is not only safe but iron in the cord blood is beneficial for the infant. Waiting for 3 minutes to clamp the cord is now recommended. This gives time for the cord blood that carries iron to be transferred to the infant. Infants have been shown to have fewer problems with anemia which strains the heart and potentially can lead to less oxygenated blood in the body. The extra cord blood is especially important for preterm newborns who receive less iron from the mother during pregnancy since they are born earlier. Low iron is associated with learning delays, sleep difficulties, poor attention, and slow growth so avoiding these problems is important.

Vitamin K

To prevent hemorrhagic disease of the newborn, infants are given a vitamin K injection after birth. Infants are at increased risk for vitamin K deficiency because it is not passed well through the placenta. In most countries, infants are given 1 mg of vitamin K by injection. An option for women concerned about any injections because of preservatives is to use oral vitamin K in the dose of 2 mgs within 6 hours of delivery and then another 2 mgs orally 1 week later. I support either option with my patients, although research has only been done on the injection form as an effective method to prevent bleeding. I recommend that all infants receive at least one form of vitamin K.

Antibiotic eye drops

Another long-standing practice after delivery is the placement of antibiotic drops into an infant's eyes. This practice began as an effort to prevent the passage of sexually transmitted diseases from the mother to the infant during delivery, such as gonorrhea or chlamydia. However, women are normally checked for these infections during prenatal care. If they do not have these infections, their infants are not susceptible and therefore the antibiotic drops are not needed. Even scheduled C-section babies receive the drops even though they do not pass through the vaginal canal and have no risk of infection. As long as a woman's medical history is negative for these infections, antibiotic drops do not need to be given. These drops can cause allergic reactions and are a source of unnecessary antibiotics.

Hepatitis B vaccine

Hepatitis B vaccine is routinely given to newborns within the first 1 to 2 days of birth. Hepatitis B can be a serious infection that causes chronic problems with the liver leading to liver failure and liver cancer. Hepatitis B is passed by blood-contaminated needles from IV drug use and by sexual transmission—neither of which I have ever seen a newborn engage in. Thus, a newborn is not at risk of exposure unless their mother carries the infection and passes it to them during delivery. All women in the U.S. with prenatal care are screened for infections from hepatitis B. If they are positive, their newborn infants are given a different stronger vaccine and a blood solution that gives the infants extra immune protection from the infection. As long as a woman's hepatitis B status is negative, vaccination for hepatitis B is not medically necessary following birth. The vaccine may challenge or compromise the infant's immune system that is very immature at birth. Many children with autism have compromised immune systems. No studies have proven that immunity for hepatitis B develops after vaccination following birth and whether this immunity is maintained to early adulthood when it would be important. Parents and their doctor should make the decision as to whether a baby should be inoculated after birth for hepatitis B based upon the individual risks and benefits to the child.

Summary

Preconception and pregnancy practices described in previous chapters give a woman the best chance of having a normal delivery. Even with the best preparation, the delivery of an infant is an unpredictable event. Some decisions can be made in advance; other decisions need to be made quickly. By understanding and discussing delivery practices, options, and decisions with their doctor or midwife, women can make the best decisions for their own health and for the best short- and long-term health outcome of their new child.

CHAPTER 17 REFERENCES

1. Bilder D, Pinborough-Zimmerman J, Miller J, McMahon W. Prenatal, perinatal, and neonatal factors associated with autism spectrum disorders. *Pediatrics.* 2009 May;123(5):1293-300. DH389.

2. Gardener H, Spiegelman D. Buka S, Prenatal risk factors for autism: comprehensive meta-analysis, *British Journal of Psychiatry.* 2009 Jul;195(1):7-14. DH237.

3. Glasson EJ, Bower C, Petterson B, de Klerk N, Chaney G, Hallmayer JF. Perinatal factors and the development of autism – a population study. *Arch Gen Psychiatry.* 2004 Jun;61(6):618-27. DH238.

4. Guinchat V, Thorsen P, Laurent C, Cans C, Bodeau N, Cohen D. Pre-, peri- and neonatal risk factors for autism. *Acta Obstet Gynecol Scand.* 2012 Mar;91(3):287-300. DH553.

5. Hultman CM, Sparen P, Cnattinguis S. Perinatal risk factors for infantile autism. *Epidemiology.* 2002 Jul;13(4):417-23. DH239.

6. Kolevzon A, Gross R, Reichenberg A. Prenatal and perinatal risk factors for autism: a review and integration of findings. *Arch Pediatr Adolesc Med.* 2007 Apr;161(4):326-33. DH240.

7. Langridge AT, Glasson EJ, Nassar N, Jacoby P, Pennell C, Hagan R, Bourke J, Leonard H, Stanley FJ. Maternal conditions and perinatal characteristics associated with autism spectrum disorder and intellectual disability. *PLoS One.* 2013;8(1):e50963. DH550.

8. Visser JC, Rommelse N, Vink L, Schrieken M, Oosterling IJ, van der Gaag RJ, Buitelaar JK. Narrowly Versus Broadly Defined Autism Spectrum Disorders: Differences in Pre- and Perinatal Risk Factors. *J Autism Dev Disord.* 2012 Oct 18. DH551.

9. Williams K, Helmer M, Duncan GW, Peat JK, Mellis CM. Perinatal and maternal risk factors for autism spectrum disorders in New South Wales, Australia, *Child Care Health Dev,* 2008 Mar;34(2):249-56. PMID:18257794. DH242.

10. Zhang X, Lv CC, Tian J, Miao RJ, Xi W, Hertz-Picciotto I, Qi L. Prenatal and perinatal risk factors for autism in China, *J Autism Dev Disord.* 2010 Nov;40(11):1311-21. DH243.

11. Glasson 2004.

12. Kurth L, Haussmann R. Perinatal Pitocin as an early ADHD biomarker: neurodevelopmental risk? *J Atten Disord,* 2011 Jul;15(5):423-31. DH235.

13. Alderberth I. Factors influencing the establishment of the intestinal microbiota in infancy. *Nestle Nutr Workshop Ser Pediatr Program.* 2008;62:13-33. DH50.

14. Biasucci G, Benenati B, Morelli L, Bessi E, Boehm G. Cesarean delivery may affect the early biodiversity of intestinal bacteria. *J Nutr.* 2008;138(9):1796S-1800S. DH55.

15. Grönlund MM, Lehtonen OP, Eerola E, Kero P. Fecal microflora in healthy infants born by different methods of delivery: permanent changes in intestinal flora after cesarean delivery. *J Pediatr Gastroenterol Nutr.* 1999;28(1):19-25. DH65.

16. MacKay DF, Smith GCS, Dobbie R, Pell JP. Gestational age at delivery and special educational need: retrospective cohort study of 407,503 schoolchildren. *PLoS Med.* 2010 7(6): e1000289. doi:10.1371/journal.pmed.1000289. DH555.

17. Dozier AM, Howard CR, Brownell EA, Wissler RN, Glantz JC, Ternullo SR, Thevenet-Morrison KN, Childs CK, Lawrence RA. Labor epidural anesthesia, obstetric factors and breastfeeding cessation. *Matern Child Health J.* 2012 Jun 13. DH556.

Part 4

Infancy and Early Childhood
Autism & ADHD Prevention

18

Preventative Nutrition

The goal of this entire book has been to give women the tools to have a healthy child free of autism and ADHD. The foundation is the Triangle of Prevention where the areas of nutrition, digestion, and toxins are addressed for optimal health of the mother and her child. For infants, we revisit the first cornerstone of the triangle: healthy diet and nutrition. Just as it is impossible to be healthy and have a good pregnancy without nutritious food, it is also extremely difficult to raise a healthy child with a poor diet.

Role of Nutrition in Autism

What role does nutrition play in the development of autism? My clinical experience, and that of other autism practitioners, is that most children with autism are nutritionally depleted. They have limited diets, often consisting of simple carbohydrates such as bread and pasta or dairy foods. They lack the proper levels of key vitamins, minerals, and proteins needed for proper cellular function and body growth. Essential fats such as DHA needed for neurological development and brain function are inadequate.

Since nutrition is the first part of the Triangle of Prevention, my
treatment of children with autism begins with diet analysis and nutrition evaluation. When these nutritional deficits are corrected, the
health of the child with autism improves.

Newborn Feeding

Only two choices exist to provide the entire nutritional needs of
a newborn infant: breastfeeding or formula. There are many specific
nutrients and other factors involved, so mothers need education and
support in how to best use each of these methods.

Breastfeeding

The American Academy of Pediatrics recommends breastfeeding
newborn infants and that breast milk be the only recommended food
for the first 6 months of life. Research shows that breastfeeding has a
protective effect against the development of autism[1,2,3] (formula feeding with the addition of the essential fats, DHA, and arachidonic acid
is also protective but to a lesser extent than sole breastfeeding). It is
thought that the DHA and essential fats in breast milk play a protective
role. This is consistent with the fact that essential fats are vital for brain
growth. The initial breast milk, called *colostrum*, contains protective antibodies including IgA, which help protect the infant from infections,
and also helps the initial development of their immune and digestive
systems.

A breastfeeding woman requires an extra 500 calories per day more
than a non-pregnant woman. Not eating enough following delivery and
losing weight too quickly will limit a new mother's ability to breastfeed.
The mother also needs to have increased fluid intake during breastfeeding. At least three quarts of fluid a day are recommended.

A lactating woman also needs more nutrients such as protein, iron,
calcium, and magnesium. Higher doses of vitamins A and C are also
needed, but some nutrient needs decrease such as folic acid. Adequate
intakes of essential fats, especially omega-3 fats such as DHA, are absolutely essential for proper neurologic development of the baby.

Nursing mother's diet needs (daily)

- Foods: organic when possible
- Fluids: three quarts of fluid (water, juice, or milk)
- Calories: extra 500
- Protein: 65 to 90 grams
- Vitamin C foods: at least two servings
- Green vegetables: at least two servings
- Other vegetables: at least two servings
- Eggs: one to two servings (a good brain food which has cholesterol, vitamin E, choline, sometimes DHA, and absorbable protein)
- Meats (if eaten): two to three servings
- Dairy foods (if eaten): five to six servings
- Beans: one to two servings (more if vegetarian or non-dairy diet)
- Whole grain complex carbohydrates: five servings

Nursing mother's supplement needs (daily)

- Prenatal vitamin
- DHA: 1000 mg
- Cod liver oil: one teaspoon
- Probiotic: 20 billion CFUs multi-strain with bifidus and acidophilus
- Vitamin D: 2,000 IUs in the summer or 4,000 IUs winter (or based on vitamin D level)
- Calcium: 800 to 1000 mg a day if no dairy, 400 mg with dairy
- Magnesium: 200 to 400 mg
- Zinc: 15 mg
- Vitamin C: 500 to 1000 mg
- Trace minerals: liquid or capsule
- For known positive MTHFR genetic test: methylfolate 800 mcg and methyl B12 200 mcg

Vitamin D Supplementation for Breastfed Infants

From birth, the American Academy of Pediatrics recommends that all breastfed infants be supplemented with vitamin D 400 IUs daily. The basis for this recommendation comes from the fact that breast milk has inadequate levels of vitamin D, leading to deficiencies in infants. Without adequate levels of vitamin D, the baby can develop *rickets*: a softening of the bones leading to fractures and deformities. A classic sign of rickets is a baby with severely bowed legs.

Increased rates of autism are coincident with doctors' recommendations for reduced sun exposure and the resulting lowered vitamin D levels.[4] Recommendations for sun avoidance have been overblown since the risks from brief sun exposure for most people are minimal and sunlight is required for natural vitamin D production in the body.

The primary reason vitamin D in breast milk is low is because pregnant and nursing women in the U.S. have low vitamin D levels. In the past, doctors recommended women supplement with 400 IUs/day of vitamin D during pregnancy and lactation. However, research found that this recommendation was inadequate, and 4,000 IUs/day was needed to obtain normal vitamin D levels for both the mother and a nursing infant.[5] An intake of 6,400 IUs/day was also found to be safe and free of toxicity. I recommend nursing mothers have 10 to 15 minutes of direct sunlight per day. If sunlight is unavailable, they should take 2,000 IUs in the summer or 4,000 IUs in the winter. All breastfed infants should receive 400 IUs of vitamin D daily.

Adequate Breast Milk Supply

If a woman has problems with her breast milk supply, she should work with a lactation specialist. Most midwives are excellent breastfeeding coaches as well. This can make a significant difference in establishment and maintenance of successful breastfeeding.

Stress can reduce milk supply. Every new mother is under stress with the challenging transition to parenthood. Therefore, additional help from family members, friends, or health professionals should be set up ahead of time.

There are several ways to combat a low milk supply. My first recommendation is usually to obtain a hospital-grade breast pump such as by a brand like Medela. Breast milk production is based on demand. By pumping in between feedings the body detects that more milk is needed.

There are also some safe herbs that naturally increase supply. The herb fenugreek can be very helpful. The key with fenugreek is to take adequate amounts, which is 2 to 3 capsules (600 mg total) three times a day. It takes anywhere from 1 to 3 days to see improvement. Combination herbs for nursing exist, such as in a pregnancy tea, and can be helpful. Herbs and specific vitamins can also decrease milk supply. Excess vitamin B6 and the herb sage should be avoided for this reason.

Breastfeeding an Infant with Digestive Problems

When an infant is having digestive problems, a woman can make changes to her own diet that may improve symptoms since food proteins are passed through the breast milk. If an infant is colicky and crying for hours at a time or if they are spitting up, gassy, or having blood in their stools, these are all signs that they may be reacting to a food in their mother's diet. The first food to remove from the mother's diet is dairy foods. After dairy, the most common foods to eliminate are wheat (gluten), soy, eggs, and nuts. Other foods that may cause some mild fussiness and gas in an infant are vegetables such as broccoli, onions, and garlic, although these usually do not cause the more severe allergic reactions such as blood in the stools.

Formula Feeding

Some women choose not to breastfeed, are unsuccessful in their attempts, or they and/or their infant have health problems that preclude it. These women rely on formula to provide full nutrition for the baby. Infant formula is usually based on cow milk proteins. They can also be based on soy formula, although this is becoming less common because concentrated soy is a phytoestrogen and this may be harmful, especially to male infants. There are also formulas that contain broken-down proteins that are easier to digest. Specialized formulas also are available for children with special health needs, growth needs, or problems with allergies and digestion. Formulas now exist that are organic, but are usually cow milk-based.

After analyzing several formulas through a computerized diet program, I was surprised by some of the key nutrients that were missing in formulas. The results showed that several important fats found in breast milk were not found in standard formulas, including some essential fats such as DHA. Several formulas do contain some DHA and another essential fat called arachidonic acid but in doses that are lower compared to human breast milk.

I also looked at a formula recipe from the book *Nourishing Traditions* by Sally Fallon that discusses supplements you would add to cow's milk to make a more highly nutritious infant formula. My dietary analysis of this formula found that it was extremely close to breast milk. From this result, I began to recommend adding supplements to formulas to bring the nutrition content closer to breast milk.

Formula Supplementation

Add the following to 20 ounces of formula (use organic when possible):

- Cod liver oil: ½ teaspoon (contains DHA, EPA, vitamin A, and D) (tested mercury-free)
- Cholesterol: 125 mg (1 tablespoon of clarified butter or ghee, which contains no milk protein)
- Sunflower oil: One teaspoon (omega-6 fatty acids)
- Extra virgin olive oil: ½ teaspoon (omega-9 fatty acids)
- Coconut oil: ½ teaspoon (medium chain triglycerides and saturated fat)
- Infant probiotics: with bifidobacteria and lactobacillus
- Vitamin D: 400 IUs (if not present in the cod liver oil)
- Vitamin E: 10 mg (alpha and gamma forms of vitamin E)

Formulas for Digestive Problems

There are times when an infant appears to not be tolerating a formula. Their symptoms are similar to an infant who does not tolerate breast milk, such as reflux, spitting up, arching, excessive crying, gassiness, bloating, skin rashes, diaper rash, or green/bloody stools. This is the time to stop any cow milk based formula. Since soy based formulas are a concern because they contain phytoestrogens, I recommend an organic version that has broken-down proteins. In a minority of cases the symptoms continue and I recommend trying a formula designed for severe digestive problems and allergies.

Solid Foods

The current recommendation from the U.S. pediatric community is that mothers wait until the infant is 6 months old to begin feeding any solid foods. Solid foods are any foods that are not breast milk or formula.

The basis of this recommendation is multifold. One reason is that until the sixth month the infant's digestive system is not mature enough to digest other foods well. It is also at this point that the child needs additional minerals (especially iron and zinc), because the levels at this age are inadequate in breast milk. From my experience as a pediatrician and what is practiced in other medical traditions, such as traditional Chinese medicine, foods should be introduced slowly. Most infants are much more prone to reactions from foods. Therefore the introduction of foods should be one at a time with less allergenic but nutritious concentrated foods offered first.

My Research on Introduction of First Solid Foods

In the U.S. it is recommended that an infant's first food be a simple cereal grain such as rice. Rice, particularly the white rice used in most baby foods, has little nutrition. It has few vitamins and minerals and it must be fortified with additional iron and zinc needed for the baby. Concern has been raised about an infant's ability to properly digest grains such as rice because of low levels of the enzyme amylose. There are also concerns with arsenic in rice products.[6] Rice also does not contain any fat or protein because it is primarily a simple carbohydrate. Since breast milk is 50% fat, rice is not a good substitute in terms of calories and overall nutrition.

To evaluate which first solid food is the most nutritious, I participated in a research study for my nutrition fellowship and my Masters of Science in Public Health degree. The study hypothesis was that babies fed pureed beef would have better health than babies fed rice cereal. Beef is a natural source of iron and zinc, along with having protein and fat. We started with infants age 6 months who were exclusively breastfed. We put half of them on a diet of pureed beef and half on rice cereal as the only solid food while they continued to breastfeed. We then tracked the children's growth and neurologic development. We also measured zinc and iron levels in the blood to see if they were absorbing these minerals. We followed these infants from 6 to 12 months of age.

Results showed that the infants who ate the beef had higher and more normal levels for both zinc and iron than those who ate rice cereal. There were not any differences in development and growth. However, we determined that the babies would need to be tracked well into their second year of life to confirm this result. The higher zinc and iron levels were important because both of these minerals are needed for growth and neurologic development. We disproved a widespread belief that pureed beef is not a good initial food for infants.

Plan of Solid Food Introduction

In general it is best to begin one food at a time every 3 days to watch for reactions to the food. Organic foods should be used as much as possible.

From 6 months

- First: cooked egg yolk (good brain food—recommended daily), vegetables except nightshade vegetables (avoid tomatoes, peppers, eggplant, and avocados)
- Second: fruits (except citrus) and beans
- Third: pureed meats

From 9 months

- All vegetables
- Non-gluten grains (quinoa, millet, rice, amaranth, and gluten-free oats)
- Corn (non-GM)
- Whole milk yogurts and cheeses (if infant has no history of digestive problems or allergies)

From 12 months

- Nuts and seeds
- Soy in form of tofu, miso, and soy sauce (not concentrated soy protein or soy milk)
- Wheat and other gluten grains such as barley and rye
- Whole milk dairy products if not done at 9 months
- Citrus fruits
- Seafood

Relationship of Gluten and Casein to Autism

Within the autism community, many children are on a gluten-free (no wheat or food with the protein gluten) and casein-free (no dairy) diet. There are multiple reasons that these children are on this restricted diet. Many children on the autism spectrum have digestive issues that cause them to have problems breaking down their food. Both gluten and casein are large protein molecules that are eaten in high doses by most Americans. Removing these big proteins often alleviates digestive symptoms and widens the range of foods children will eat.

The other factor is that if gluten and casein are not properly broken-down, the incompletely broken-down protein forms cause problems on their own. The incomplete breakdown protein of gluten is called *gliadomorphin* and the incomplete protein form of casein is called *caseomorphin*. Both of these proteins act like opiate peptides in the body and cause a drug-like sedation. Children tend to crave these foods and will often refuse to eat other foods. They will become cranky when they go too long without gluten or casein. These children often appear spacey and in their own world.

Since both gluten and casein can cause problems, parents of any child who has a sibling with autism may want to avoid these foods for the first two years of life to be safe. These foods should also be avoided if the child has a pattern of any chronic digestive or allergy symptoms (such as eczema), or if the child has developmental delays.

Summary

The first few years of life are an ideal time to optimize a child's nutrition. A nutritious diet (usually including breastfeeding) provides all the nutrients needed for healthy development of the nervous system. A healthy nervous system leads to the best possible chance of a child developing normally.

CHAPTER 18 REFERENCES

1. Schultz ST, Klonoff-Cohen HS, Wingard DL, Akshoomoff NA, Macera CA, Ji M, Bacher C. Breastfeeding, infant formula supplementation, and Autistic Disorder: the results of a parent survey. *International Breastfeeding Journal.* 2006, 1:16. DH557.

2. Al-Farsi YM, Al-Sharbati MM, Waly MI, Al-Farsi OA, Al-Shafaee MA, Al-Khaduri MM, Trivedi MS, Deth RC. Effect of suboptimal breast-feeding on occurrence of autism: a case-control study. *Nutrition.* 2012 Jul;28(7-8):e27-32. DH558.

3. Burd L, Fisher W, Kerbeshian J, Vesely B, Durgin B, Reep P. A comparison of breastfeeding rates among children with pervasive developmental disorder, and controls. *J Dev Behav Pediatr.* 1988 Oct;9(5):247-51. DH559.

4. Cannell JJ. Autism and vitamin D. *Med Hypotheses.* 2008;70(4):750-9. DH463.

5. Basile LA, Taylor SN, Wagner CL, Horst RL, Hollis BW. The effect of high-dose vitamin D supplementation on serum vitamin D levels and milk calcium concentration in lactating women and their infants. *Breastfeed Med.* 2006 Spring;1(1):27-35. DH464.

6. Hite AH. Arsenic and rice: A call for regulation. *Nutrition.* 2013 Jan:29(1);353-4. DH560.

19

Building Healthy Immune and Digestive Systems

Strong digestion is the second cornerstone of the Triangle of Prevention. Once good food is consumed, the child's body must be able to digest and absorb the food. Without a strong digestive system, their body will not take in adequate nutrients—no matter how healthy the food.

A strong digestive system is also integral to a strong immune system—one cannot build one without the other. Approximately 70% of our immune system is harbored within the walls of the digestive system. Any foreign substance, such as bacteria, that enters our body with food comes into direct contact with our immune system. Thus, the immune cells in our digestive system are one of the body's first lines of defense.

Role of Immune and Digestion Problems in Autism and ADHD

A consensus paper released from the American Academy of Pediatrics in 2010, summarized research on gastrointestinal problems of children with autism and found that the prevalence may be as high as 70%.[1,2] The severity of the gastrointestinal problems correlated with the severity of the autism symptoms.[3] In my practice, I find that the majority of children with autism have some type of digestive problem. These digestive issues include gastroesophageal reflux, esophagitis, abdominal pain, diarrhea, constipation, irritable bowel syndrome, and inflammatory bowel disease such as Crohn's disease and ulcerative colitis. Understanding the association between digestion problems and autism has led to a significant step forward in treating these children. While these digestive issues are very common with autism, they can also be problems in children with ADHD, although not as often or as severe.

My first line of treatment for children with autism and ADHD is always to address nutritional problems. After addressing these deficiencies, my next step is to identify and treat digestive problems. This often includes treatment of dysbiosis (improper types or levels of gut flora) in the intestine, healing the intestine, and strengthening immune function. These therapies help decrease inflammation and improve health and functioning of these children.

Development of the Immune and Digestive Systems

An important strategy in preventing autism and ADHD is to help the newborn/infant develop strong digestion and immune systems. Nature has designed two ways for an infant to develop their digestive and immune system.

The first way for this to occur is through the ingestion of healthy bacteria during a vaginal delivery.[4,5] These healthy bacteria, such as lactobacillus, populate the digestive tract of the infant and prime the immune system. The immune system then develops the ability to distinguish between substances that cause infection, such as bacteria, and substances that do not, such as food. Children without good bacteria often develop digestive symptoms, such as reflux or diarrhea, and immune problems, such as recurrent infections and allergies.

The second way for the development of the digestive and the immune systems is through breast milk. Breast milk contains proteins, antibodies, and enzymes that help the infant fight infections. These substances also help the infant better digest and absorb the nutrients they need from their food.

Supporting a Healthy Immune System

Since probiotics and breast milk are two cornerstones for the development of the digestive system, they are also the foundation for building a healthy immune system. Breastfeeding for the first one to two years of life is one of the best things a mother can do for her child's health. Since anything a mother consumes or is exposed to will pass through her breast milk, this breast milk will be most beneficial coming from a mother with good nutrition and minimal toxins.

The addition of probiotics for both the mother and child is essential for the development of a healthy immune system. I recommend supplementing all infants with a probiotic designed specifically for that age group. It should contain both bifidus and lactobacillus bacteria. Nursing mothers should also consume a probiotic designed for women on a daily basis. Cultured foods such as kefir are a good addition to the mother's diet.

For additional immune support, there are some specific vitamins and minerals that help support a child's immune system. These are especially important if a child has a lot of exposure to people with illnesses or they are getting sick frequently. Table 19.1 below has immune support recommendations for children over the age of one year. For children from 6 to 12 months, I recommend homeopathic vitamin C tablets and 5 mg of zinc given with food. The essential oils in this table can be used at any age but, the smaller the child, the smaller the dose that should be used.

Because of their potency, essential oils should only be used with babies and young children under the direction of a trained practitioner. Essential oils are anti-bacterial, anti-viral, and/or anti-inflammatory, depending on the type. Some of these essential oils also support immune function. These oils include tea tree oil, eucalyptus radiata, thyme linolol, lavender, and Roman chamomile, individually or in a blend. Either diffuse these oils or mix one to two drops in one tablespoon of olive oil and place on the child's chest.

Table 19.1 - General Immune Support: Acute Treatment at the Beginning of an Infection (Age 12 Months and Older)

Category	Supplement	Dose	Frequency
Vitamin	Vitamin A	2500 IUs	1 time a day
	Bioflavonoids	150 mg	1 time a day
	Vitamin C	50 mg x age of child in years	2 times a day
Mineral	Zinc	15 mg	1 time a day

Medicines of Concern

There are two medicines frequently used in children that can lead to the development of digestive problems: antibiotics and stomach acid blockers. Sometimes they are absolutely necessary, yet in many cases they are overused or given for too long a time period, creating digestive and eventually immune problems. Studies have begun to explore the link between autism and antibiotics.[6,7] It is my clinical experience that children with autism and children with digestive problems often have had extensive treatments with antibiotics and/or acid blockers.

Avoiding Excess Antibiotics

Antibiotics can trigger a series of events that lead to long-term deterioration of children's digestive and immunity systems. One study found that gut flora remained disturbed for four years following antibiotics.[8]

Example of how antibiotics can lead to health problems

A young child is treated with antibiotics. The antibiotics disrupt the normal good bacteria in the intestine. If the good probiotic bacteria are not restored, opportunistic bacteria and yeast grow and cause an imbalance of organisms, called dysbiosis, in the intestine. Dysbiosis leads to the development of multiple digestive symptoms. The child develops diarrhea or constipation, or a pattern of alternating digestive problems called irritable bowel syndrome. Since disrupting the digestive system also disrupts the immune system, the dysbiosis becomes chronic and the child develops food allergies and sensitivities to foods. These allergies and sensitivities lead to symptoms seen anywhere in the body such as eczema, stomach pain, and respiratory symptoms.

Antibiotics only treat bacterial infections. They do not treat viral infections—the most common type of infection in children. Early in the course of a child's illness it can be difficult to determine whether the infection is viral or bacterial. Rather than prescribing antibiotics early in the illness, for most illnesses the child should be closely monitored by the parents under the care of their physician. Should the symptoms indicate a bacterial infection, then an antibiotic may be warranted. However in most cases, the symptoms will develop consistent with a viral infection and no antibiotics are needed. This one change of practice could dramatically reduce the use of antibiotics in this country and greatly improve the functioning of the digestive systems of our children. Close monitoring of the child with a knowledgeable health care practitioner and educated parents can often avoid the use of unnecessary antibiotics.

Antibiotics can be life saving and there are times when they need to be used in young children. Should they be necessary, it is important to supplement the child with higher doses of probiotics during and after the course of antibiotics. Research shows that it may take up to three months after the use of antibiotics to restore the good bacteria. I recommend a broad-spectrum probiotic with a combination of multiple strains of bifidus and lactobacillus. If the child is under one year of age, I recommend an infant formula with probiotics. For children over one year, adult doses of 10 billion colony-forming units are readily available and are safe. Probiotic treatment following use of antibiotics should be at twice the maintenance dose. Should there be any digestive symptoms during the course of antibiotic treatment, the dose of probiotics should be increased.

Avoiding the Use of Acid Blockers

The other medicine overused in children is acid blockers. Medicines that block stomach acid are often used for gastroesophageal reflux and relieving colicky symptoms in infants. Many infants spit up after feeding partly because the muscles controlling the passage from the esophagus to the stomach are immature. If stomach acid comes up into the esophagus, it can cause pain often seen in symptoms of colic. Acid blocking medicines, such as Zantac and Prilosec, prevent the formation of acid in the stomach. They do not actually stop the food from coming up the esophagus, or prevent the infant from spitting up after feeding.

Stomach acid has several important digestive functions. The first is that it breaks down proteins. Without the acid, proteins in food such as casein in milk are passed intact further into the intestines. The immune system in the intestines cannot process an intact casein protein; therefore it reacts to it as a foreign substance. Since it is considered a foreign substance, the immune system mounts an attack where antibodies against the food develop, leading to food allergies and sensitivities.

The acid in the stomach is also meant as a first line immune defense against bacteria and other pathogens that arrive in the stomach with food. If the acid doesn't kill these pathogens, they travel further into the intestines where they can cause an imbalance or dysbiosis. Dysbiosis, as explained above, leads to many different kinds of digestive problems.

Acid in the stomach is also a signal for the digestive system to release bicarbonate to buffer the acid as it travels through the digestive system. The body is signaled to release other digestive hormones that help break down carbohydrates. It is easy to see how the use of this one type of medicine can disrupt a cascade of normal digestive processes leading to chronic digestive problems, malabsorption, food allergies, and sensitivities. This is a pattern I see frequently in children with autism and in other children with digestive problems. Along with this pattern, I often see the development of recurrent infections, such as ear infections, from a weakened immune system. Pediatricians often treat these infections with more antibiotics causing a cycle of health decline. In the next section, I describe natural treatments for reflux that do not block stomach acid, but can provide relief to infants.

It should be noted that some children with neurologic or muscular diseases with low muscle tone have severe reflux. These children will often truly benefit from use of acid blocker medications. The use of natural treatments and monitoring of digestion is still important.

Treatment of Specific Digestive Issues
Colic, intestinal gas, stomach pain, gastroesophageal reflux, and spitting up

All infants will cry and be fussy at times. The vast majority will also spit up some breast milk or formula. Concern arises when an infant is repeatedly fussy and uncomfortable after eating. A classic sign of a medical concern is if they are more uncomfortable when lying down and when they arch their back and cry.

There are adjustments that can be made to a mother's diet if she is nursing that may help. The first is to begin probiotics for both the mother and her infant. The next is to eliminate all dairy products from the mother's diet including cheese, cow milk, yogurt, and ice cream for a few days to see if that helps. Sometimes eliminating one type of food such as dairy will help clear up many of these issues. If this does not help, then the mother should begin an elimination diet by taking out the most common allergenic foods, which are dairy, gluten grains (wheat), soy, eggs, and nuts.

As stated in the last chapter, if the infant is formula-fed, switching from cow milk-based formula to a formula with broken-down proteins may be helpful. I do not recommend a soy protein, which can also be difficult to digest. If these formulas are not helpful, sometimes a specialized formula for digestive problems and allergies is helpful.

Natural treatments also exist. A classic is something called *gripe water* that can be obtained even in regular pharmacies. It is a combination of gentle herbs for gas such as chamomile. The medicine *simethicone* is a safe over-the-counter product that stays in the digestive tract and eliminates gas. I use essential oils in my practice and some blends of essential oils can be used during stomach massage on infants. Finally, craniosacral or osteopathic adjustment of an infant by a qualified practitioner can make a big difference in calming a colicky infant and helping reduce reflux.

Diarrhea

The best treatment for chronic diarrhea is to determine the cause. This may entail looking for reactions to foods or dysbiosis. An elimination diet for determining food reactions can be helpful, or a health care practitioner can evaluate for food allergies and sensitivities.

Almost all young children will at some point suffer from diarrhea. Most bouts are short-lived and caused by a food or a virus. Unless diarrhea is from identified bacteria, antibiotics are not needed and may in fact worsen symptoms.

Since dehydration is the primary concern from diarrhea, attention should be given to restoring fluids. The best fluid for a young child is breast milk with the addition of a specially formulated electrolyte solution for children. Older children should use the classic diet for acute diarrhea called the *BRAT diet* which consists of Bananas, Rice, Applesauce, and Toast along with an electrolyte drink.

The probiotic yeast called *saccharomyces boulardii* has been shown to be helpful for shortening the course of acute diarrheal illness or from antibiotic-associated diarrhea. One to two capsules of a 3 to 5 billion colony forming units strength is a good daily dose.

Constipation

With the Standard American Diet (SAD) of low fiber and high-sugar foods, constipation is quite common. Therefore, improving the diet is a logical first step. Treatment should begin by increasing fruits, vegetables, and complex carbohydrates with fiber. It is helpful to avoid constipating foods, such as bananas and rice, used to treat diarrhea. Dairy products should be reduced, as they are also a frequent cause of constipation in children. Drinking adequate fluids is also important.

It is helpful to supplement the diet changes with probiotics (combination of acidophilus and bifidus). I also recommend adding healthy fats to the diet: cod liver oil, olive oil, and flax seed oil. Additional magnesium and vitamin C are also helpful for constipation. For children, 100 mg of magnesium at night is helpful for constipation, as well as calming the child and promoting sleep.

Summary

Developing and maintaining a healthy digestive system is important for the prevention of autism. Ideally, women should begin this before conception so they can give their babies a healthy start during delivery. If an infant receives good bacteria along with healthy breast milk, the digestive and immune systems will begin to develop normally. Probiotic and formula supplementation are important additions if needed. Finally, the judicious use of antibiotics and acid blockers can go a long way toward preventing disruptions of digestive and immune functions.

CHAPTER 19 REFERENCES

1. Buie T, et al. Evaluation, diagnosis and treatment of gastrointestinal disorders in individuals with ASDs: a consensus report. *Pediatrics.* 2010;125(suppl 1):S1-S18. DH56.

2. Valincenti-McDermott M, McVicar K, Rapin I, Wershil BK, Cohen H, Shinnar S. Frequency of gastrointestinal symptoms in children with autistic spectrum disorders and association with family history of autoimmune disease. *J Dev Behav Pediatr.* 2006;27(2 suppl):S128-136. DH85.

3. Adams JB, Johansen L, Powell L, Quig D, Rubin R. Gastrointestinal flora and gastrointestinal status in children with autism -- comparisons to typical children and correlation with autism severity. *BMC Gastroenterol.* 2011;11:22. DH380.

4. Biasucci G, Benenati B, Morelli L, Bessi E, Boehm G. Cesarean delivery may affect the early biodiversity of intestinal bacteria. *J Nutr.* 2008;138(9):1796S-1800S. DH55.

5. Buie T, et al. Evaluation, diagnosis and treatment of gastrointestinal disorders in individuals with ASDs: a consensus report. *Pediatrics.* 2010;125(suppl 1):S1-S18. DH56.

6. Fallon J. Could one of the most widely prescribed antibiotics amoxicillin/clavulanate "augmentin" be a risk factor for autism? *Med Hypotheses.* 2005;64(2):312-5. DH561.

7. Manev R, Manev H. Aminoglycoside antibiotics and autism: a speculative hypothesis. *BMC Psychiatry.* 2001;1:5. DH562.

8. Jakobsson HE, Jernberg C, Andersson AF, Sjölund-Karlsson M, Jansson JK, et al. (2010) Short-Term Antibiotic Treatment Has Differing Long-Term Impacts on the Human Throat and Gut Microbiome. *PLoS ONE* 5(3): e9836. doi:10.1371/journal.pone.0009836. DH566.

20

Non-Toxic Children

In order to attain our goal of having healthy children, we must ensure the safety of their environment. Healthy children are non-toxic children. Since children are small with immature body organs, they are at high risk for adverse reactions. Any chemical that is dangerous when a woman is pregnant is also dangerous for a young child.

The avoidance of toxins is the focus in the third part of the Triangle of Prevention. Our goal with this chapter is to review sources of common childhood toxins and how to avoid exposure. These toxins can be in anything a child eats or puts in their mouth. For very young children, this includes pacifiers and toys. Anything that a child touches also needs to be considered, such as their clothes, bedding, and any skin care product.

In the home environment, it is important to consider everything from what paint is used on the walls to what type of fabric is used for the furniture. In this chapter, I want to bring awareness, not fear or paranoia. Women and young children are all exposed to toxins, so the goal is to remove as many as possible and make sure their detoxification systems are as strong as possible.

Role of Environmental Toxins in Autism and ADHD

An ever-increasing number of research articles show the detrimental effects of chemicals in our environment on developing children, beginning in utero.[1,2,3,4] Many of these chemicals harm the development of the nervous system and lead to the neurological issues seen in children with autism and ADHD. Toxins also disrupt the energy pathways of the cell in the mitochondria and harm the body's natural ability to detoxify. Exposure to toxins is part of the development of autism and ADHD, and ongoing exposure plays a role in the maintenance of symptoms. Helping these children improve their body's detoxification systems and minimizing ongoing toxin exposure improves their health.

When I treat children with autism and ADHD, improving detoxification ability and detoxifying are my third line of treatment after nutritional support and healing the digestive and immune systems.

Skin Care

Just as there are many chemicals in cosmetics and makeup products used by adults, there are also many in products marketed for infants. These include baby oils, lotions, bubble bath, soaps, shampoos, and diaper creams. Ingredients of concern include many of the preservatives, such as parabens, discussed before. Avoiding parabens and phthalates that can act as hormone disruptors makes good sense. Any product based on petroleum is not beneficial and potentially harmful. Baby oil is mineral oil from petroleum with added artificial fragrance. This product contains a double dose of harm from the fragrance and the petroleum in a nonessential product.

In addition to the concern with harmful ingredients listed on the product label is the possibility of the product containing contaminants not listed. In 2009, The Campaign for Safe Cosmetics tested 48 infant and young child skin care products for the contaminants formaldehyde and 1,4-dioxane.[5] Both of these toxins can be produced when preservatives commonly used in these products break down. The results showed 82% of products contained formaldehyde, 67% contained 1,4-dioxane, and 61% contained both. It is appalling that products marketed for the sensitive skin of children are contaminated with toxic chemicals. To avoid possible contamination with formaldehyde, women should look for and avoid ingredients such as quaternium-15, DMDM hydantoin, imidazolidinyl urea and diazolidinyl urea.

The ingredient 1,4-dioxane is a byproduct of ethoxylation where ingredients are processed with ethylene oxide. Common ingredients likely to be contaminated with 1,4-dioxane include PEG-100 stearate, sodium laureth sulfate, polyethylene, and ceteareth-20. It is easy for child care product companies to remove the toxic contaminants but they are not required to do so.

The truth is that an infant does not need all of these specialized skin products. In fact, a bath with a simple soap about one to two times a week is all that is needed. Regularly using a multitude of products with many ingredients is not necessary. Parents are putting products on an infant's skin that they do not need, with chemicals that are harmful. It does not make sense. Less is easier, cheaper, and most importantly, safer.

Healthy Options for Skin Care

For easy skin care, the baby only needs organic single-ingredient oils, a few essential oils, a few hydrosols (or flower waters), and basic unscented glycerine soap. This is much easier than buying multiple products with multiple ingredients, which greatly increases toxin exposure.

For essential oils, parents should follow the advice of a practitioner trained in their use. Essential oils are the pure oils from plants without any chemicals added. When an herb such as lavender is distilled, it is broken-down into two constituents, the essential oil and the hydrosol, both of which are great natural products to use on a child.

I find these essential oils and their hydrosol counterparts wonderful for skin care, treating infections, helping with sleep, and for cleaning, among other uses. Parents should be careful when searching for essential oils because they should only use an organic product from a reputable company. If the product label mentions fragrance or any ingredient other than the proper name of the plant, then it is not a pure oil.

Different oils have different strengths and parents need to know what oils are safe to use at specific ages. An excellent reference all about essential oils is *The Complete Book of Essential Oils and Aromatherapy* by Valerie Worwood. It is important never to put an essential oil directly on the skin of a child. Since hydrosols are water based, they are safe to use alone. A few drops of an essential oil are used with a tablespoon of a base oil. For an infant, I only recommend adding one to two drops of an essential oil to a base oil.

Essential oils

Important notes: (1) Use under the direction of a qualified medical practitioner, (2) never put essential oils directly on the baby's skin

- Newborns: Roman chamomile and lavender
- After 6 months: the above plus mandarin, eucalyptus, tea tree, thyme linolol, ravensara, and calendula

Base oils (oils to mix with essential oils)

- Newborns: sweet almond, borage, olive, calendula, and shea butter
- After six months: the above plus safflower, sunflower, coconut, grapeseed, jojoba, and avocado

Hydrosols

Roman chamomile is the primary hydrosol I recommend for diaper rash, a clogged tear duct, or irritated skin. It can also be used to make diaper wipes.

Soaps and shampoos

Glycerine soap mixed with one drop of lavender or chamomile can be used for safe cleaning of an infant.

Clothing, Bedding, and Mattresses

One of the biggest toxin concerns with fabric in clothing, bedding, and mattresses is that they often have been manufactured with fire retardant chemicals called *PBDEs (polybrominated diphenyl ethers)*. These include the fabric coverings in car seats, baby carriers, and strollers.

These products are in direct contact with a child's skin that will absorb any chemical placed on it. These chemicals also off-gas fumes which are inhaled by the infant.

The PBDEs harm the developing nervous system and alter thyroid hormone function. Research in animals has shown the chemicals will induce problems with hyperactivity, learning, and memory, along with disruption of the T4 thyroid hormone.[6] A common source of flame retardants is mattresses. Children spend many hours sleeping and therefore they have the potential for a high dose of exposure from their mattresses. Buying an organic mattress is a good health investment. I have wondered whether the reduction in SIDS (Sudden Infant Death Syndrome) is because children are inhaling less toxic fumes by sleeping on their backs.

The majority of materials used for bedding and pajamas are made of polyester and cotton blends. If clothing or bedding has polyester fiber it contains plastic, which is made from petroleum. These products can also be labeled "wrinkle resistant," which means additional chemicals are used on the fabric—often including the carcinogen formaldehyde. All of these synthetic and chemically treated fabrics can off-gas toxic fumes and should be avoided. The best fabrics are 100% organic cotton, bamboo, hemp, linen, or wool. Since any detergent used on clothes or bedding will come into contact with the child's skin, avoiding conventionally scented detergents and fabric softeners is important.

Diapers and Wipes

Infants and young toddlers will be almost constantly in diapers. This is a large exposure directly on the skin. There are really only two diaper options: disposable or cloth.

Disposable diapers contain three primary layers: a plastic outer layer, a super-absorbent chemical middle layer, and an inner liner. Sodium polyacrylate is a commonly used absorbent chemical in the middle part of the diaper and it can cause allergic reactions. Disposable diapers can also contain dyes and dioxin as by-products of chlorine bleaching. Volatile organic chemicals (VOCs) such as toluene, xylene, ethylbenzene, and dipentene can also be released from disposable diapers.[7] All of these chemicals are toxic to developing nervous systems with long-term exposure. Finally, there is a large environmental impact from disposing of these diapers with toxic chemicals.

Newer disposable diapers are available that are made with fewer chemicals and without chlorine. Parents should buy these safer disposable diapers if they use disposable diapers for their baby.

Cotton diapers are available but there are also safety concerns. It is important to choose diapers made from organic cotton to avoid pesticide exposure. People can buy their own diapers or use a diaper service that washes the diapers. The primary concern with a diaper service is the fact that they need to use bleach to sanitize the diapers. With bleach, the infant will be exposed to the toxic chemical chlorine along with its potentially dangerous by-products.

Baby wipes can also contain many unsafe ingredients. These are used frequently in direct contact with an infant's skin for years so they should be as safe as possible. Harmful ingredients include alcohol, perfume, chlorine bleach, and dioxin as a by-product. Safer alternatives exist. I usually recommend a homemade wipe with Roman chamomile hydrosol on clean organic cotton. Commercially-available baby wipes with safer and more natural ingredients are available. Simple and safe is a good combination.

Pacifiers

By calming a fussy infant, pacifiers can be helpful for both the infant and their parents. Since they go in the mouth, they need to be as toxin-free as possible. Pacifiers are usually made from either latex rubber or silicone. Latex rubber should be avoided for several reasons. Latex can cause allergic reactions, including serious reactions such as anaphylaxis. They also break down more quickly than silicone and can release volatile carcinogenic chemicals called *nitrosamines*.[8] As they break down they may also harbor bacteria. Silicone is the better choice.

Bottles, Nipples, and Cups

Infants and young children use an assortment of baby bottles with nipples and sippy cups. These are meant to be sturdy and not easily broken, yet they go into a child's mouth so they need to be made from safe materials. Nipples for baby bottles are usually made from latex rubber or silicone. Just like pacifiers, silicone is the better choice. Bottles and cups are often made from plastic. The primary concerns with plastic are the types of plastic used. Avoiding BPA and phthalates used in plastics is very important for the health of the baby. There is a lot more awareness recently of the dangers of BPA so it is important for all of these products to say they are "BPA-free" right on the package. Glass bottles are available and are the safest choice.

Toys

In 2007, the potential for toys to be a source of toxins came to the forefront when over a million toy trains were pulled from the market for high levels of lead in the paint.[9] This led to the development of the 2008 U.S. Consumer Product Safety Improvement Act (CPSIA) that amended the Consumer Product Safety Act of 1972. Although the CPSIA set stricter standards for lead and phthalate levels in toys, there is still major progress that needs to be made in order to ensure the safety of toys for our children. Once again, the E.U. is ahead of us in safety regulations for toys as well as personal care products.

Toxic chemicals in toys fall into several categories: heavy metals, phthalates, flame-retardants, azo dyes, BPA, and other plastics. The primary heavy metals in toys are lead and cadmium. Lead can be in painted toys and in children's jewelry. Unfortunately in an effort for toy manufacturers to decrease lead exposure, the use of cadmium in toy paint, metal clasps, and charms has increased. Both lead and cadmium are absorbed readily when toys are placed in a child's mouth. Flame-retardants such as PBDEs have been found in hard plastic, stuffed toys, and in soft rubber toys imported from China.[10] Azo dyes are the primary dye used in textile and leather toys. These dyes are absorbed upon contact with the skin and are carcinogenic. Luckily, BPA is becoming less common in many products targeted for children as awareness to its dangers increases.

Fortunately, awareness of toxins in toys has led to the production of eco-friendly toys made out of wood and organic cotton. A good resource for healthy toys can be found at www.healthytoys.org.

Paints and Other Indoor Pollutants

Paints are a source of a group of pollutants called volatile organic compounds or VOCs. Other decorating materials, cleaners, and office equipment such as printers emit VOCs. New carpets and furniture can also off-gas dangerous chemicals. Any indoor scent or odor often contains VOCs. These chemicals have immediate effects such as eye and nose irritation, headaches, and nausea. Long-term cumulative effects include respiratory, allergy, and immune problems in children.[11] Fortunately low- or no-VOC paints are available for decorating, especially in any room a child spends a lot of time in. Depending on sensitivity and underlying health problems, an air purifier can reduce the amount of VOCs and other pollutants in indoor air.

Summary

We know that a developing child is extremely sensitive to the harmful effects of toxins. This sensitivity begins in utero and continues well into the first several years of life. It is essential to remove, or at least reduce, children's exposure to toxins. Many people assume that if a product is marketed for a child in the U.S., it has been proven to be safe. Unfortunately, this is not the case because products are removed from the market only once they have been found to be dangerous to health. Awareness and education about childhood toxin sources and avoidance are crucial for the protection of our children.

1. Jones L, Parker JD, Mendola P. Blood lead and mercury levels in pregnant women in the United States, 2003-2008. *NCHS Data Brief.* 2010;(52):1-8. DH298.

2. Lovasi GS, Quinn JW, Rauh VA, Perera FP, Andrews HF, Garfinkel R, Hoepner L, Whyatt R, Rundle A. Chlorpyrifos exposure and urban residential environment characteristics as determinants of early childhood neurodevelopment. *Am J Public Health.* 2011 Jan;101(1):63-70. DH432.

3. EPA. Universe of Chemicals and General Validation Principles. Office of Chemical Safety & Pollution Prevention, EPA publication. *U.S. Environmental Protection Agency Endocrine Disruptor Screening Program.* 2012 Nov. DH484.

4. Wigle DT, Arbuckle TE, Turner MC, Berube A, Yang Q, Liu S, Krewski D. Epidemiologic evidence of relationships between reproductive and child health outcomes and environmental chemical contaminants. *J Toxicol Environ Health B Crit Rev.* 2008;11(5-6):373-517. DH309.

5. Sarantis H, Malkan S, Archer L. Children's Bath Products Contaminated with Formaldehyde, 1,4-Dioxane. *Campaign for Safe Cosmetics.* 2009. DH492.

6. Costa L. and Giordano G. Developmental neurotoxicity of polybrominated diphenyl ether (PBDE) flame retardants. *Neuro Tox.* 2007 (28) 1047-1067. DH148.

7. Anderson RC, Anderson JH. Acute respiratory effects of diaper emissions. *Arch Environ Health.* 1999 Sep-Oct;54(5):353-8. DH493.

8. Billedeau SM, Thompson HC Jr, Miller BJ, Wind ML. Volatile N-nitrosamines in infant pacifiers sold in the United States as determined by gas chromatography/ thermal energy analysis. *J Assoc Off Anal Chem.* 1986 Jan-Feb;69(1):31-4. DH494.

9. U.S. Consumer Product Safety Commission. RC2 Corp. recalls various Thomas & Friends wooden railway toys due to lead poisoning hazard. Release #07-212. 2007. DH496.

10. Chen SJ, Ma YJ, Wang J, Chen D, Luo XJ, Mai BX. Brominated flame retardants in children's toys: concentration, composition, and children's exposure and risk assessment. *Environ Sci Technol.* 2009 Jun 1;43(11):4200-6. DH497.

11. Mendell MJ. Indoor residential chemical emmissions as risk factors for respiratory and allergic effects in children: a review. *Indoor Air J.* 2007;17:259-77. DH490.

21

Vaccines

Vaccines are designed to protect our children from infectious diseases. It is a natural parental instinct to protect our children from illness and suffering. In the early to mid-20th century, there were many deadly diseases and diseases such as polio that could cause serious life-long disability. Vaccines were successful in wiping out many of these diseases. As a parent and a physician, there are still infectious diseases that I fear children will develop.

Today, we do not routinely see children die from infectious diseases such as diphtheria, or lose their hearing from meningitis. As the number of vaccines has increased, many of those available today are for diseases that are not life threatening. Should children develop these diseases, treatment is often not needed and the majority of children recover without complications. Because of this, people today often forget the true original purpose of vaccination: to protect from life-threatening or long-term debilitating diseases.

Since the 1960s, the vaccination program has vastly changed. Every decade has seen a significant increase in the number of vaccines.

Common vaccines such as the pertussis vaccine are now given multiple times throughout childhood, and the number of different vaccines has increased dramatically. Previously, children received vaccines only in the first several years of life. Now, vaccines are recommended throughout the life cycle: in adolescents, pregnant women, and older adults. The increase in the number and types of vaccines, along with a decrease in children dying from infectious disease, has led many to question the reasons behind our current immunization program. Concern has been fueled by the fact that during the same decades, we now have ever increasing numbers of children with chronic illness and neurological problems such as autism and ADHD. Does this correlation have a causal relationship?

In the autism community, vaccinations have become a contentious issue. There are researchers and parents of children with autism who are adamant that the vaccines are either a contributing cause or *the* cause of autism. On the other extreme are those researchers and health care providers who state there is definitive proof that no causal association exists, and vilify those that disagree. This leaves new parents to sort through the information on whether vaccination is safe for themselves and their children.

In my opinion, there needs to be much more consideration and research into the individual risk factors for vaccines. Why do some children have issues with vaccinations when the majority of children do not? We need to investigate the individual issues, whether they are genetic, immune, allergic, exposure or toxin-related. When we understand the children who are at higher risk, we have the potential to have specific vaccines and varying schedules that are safe for both the health of the individual and the general public.

How Vaccines Work

Vaccines are a medical intervention to protect people from getting a disease. To make a vaccine, a virus or bacteria is either weakened or killed. A substance is added called an *adjuvant* to increase the effectiveness of the vaccine in producing an immune response. In many vaccines today, aluminum is used as the adjuvant. Often preservatives are used to protect the vaccine from contamination.

Inoculation is the process of injecting the substance into the body. Vaccines can be delivered via injection or they can be given through the mouth or nose. The vaccine stimulates the immune system to recognize the infectious virus or bacteria and try to destroy it. By trying to destroy the virus or bacteria, the body develops an immune memory. In the future, if a person is exposed to the actual disease, the body's immune system remembers the disease and is able to fight it so the person does not develop the disease.

Current Vaccine Schedule

The vaccine schedule in the U.S. seems to be constantly changing and growing. New recommendations are made every year. Vaccination schedules also vary by country; and currently, the U.S. has the highest number of vaccines. The latest recommendations add up to 49 doses of 14 vaccines by age 6 or a total of 68 doses by the age of 18. This has steadily increased from 7 infections, 3 infections and 10 doses in 1983.

Concern has been raised about whether there is evidence that the increase in vaccinations is safe for children. The Institute of Medicine (IOM) released a report in January 2013 to address this issue called *The Childhood Immunization Schedule and Safety: Stakeholder Concerns, Scientific Evidence and Future Studies.*[1] The purpose of the report was to evaluate the scientific evidence of the current CDC recommended vaccination schedule for children ages 0 to 6 years old. Interestingly, the IOM committee pointed out more than once in the report that there was inadequate evidence supporting the current schedule. Fewer than 40 studies were published in the last 10 years to address the 0-6 year old vaccine recommendations. Since the schedule adds new vaccines, and adds additional boosters every year, there is a significant gap in our understanding of the safety of the vaccines both individually and in combination. Also, the committee identified that certain populations of people may have increased susceptibility to experience reactions to vaccines. It also cited lack of scientific evidence to determine whether or not the timing and the number of doses of vaccines were related to developmental or allergic health issues in children.

2013 Center for Disease Control Recommended Vaccine Schedule: Pregnancy through age 18 (www.cdc.gov)

1. Influenza (flu vaccine): pregnancy, twice in the first year of life and then yearly

2. Hepatitis B: birth, 1- 2 months and 6 months

3. Diptheria, tetanus, pertussis (DTaP): pregnancy, 2 months, 4 months, 6 months, 18 months, 4-6 years, 6th grade and 10th grade (given together in 1 shot)

4. Polio: 2 months, 4 months, 6 months and 4-6 years

5. Haemophilus Influenza (HIB): 2 months, 4 months, 6 months and 12-15 months

6. Rotavirus: 2 months, 4 months and 6 months

7. Pneumococcal: 2 months, 4 months, 6 months and 12-15 months

8. Measles, Mumps, Rubella (MMR): 12-15 months and 4-6 years

9. Varicella (chicken pox): 12-15 months and 4-6 years

10. Hepatitis A: two doses between 12-18 months

11. Human Papillomavirus (HPV): three doses ages 11-12 years

12. Meningococcal: 11-12 years and booster before college

Contraindications for Vaccines

The CDC has a resource guide of contraindications for vaccines. It lists the contraindications by symptom and then by specific vaccine. Notes listed on separate pages provide important information.

In general, the most significant contraindications are life-threatening allergies to any of the ingredients in vaccines, such as eggs, latex, gelatin, or penicillin. Any life-threatening reaction to a specific vaccine is a contraindication to getting a future booster shot of that vaccine. For autoimmune diseases such as Guillan-Barre, and immunodeficiency diseases such as HIV, some vaccines are contraindicated, but not all.

In addition to contraindications, there are also precautions. Precautions mean that the vaccine can still be given but does not state whether the practitioner should discuss this with a parent or whether the choice is the parent's or the practitioner's.

After reviewing the precautions, I was most interested in those listed for the DTaP vaccine (diphtheria, tetanus, pertussis) because of personal experience with my son and some nebulous words about evolving neurologic disorders. After my son's second DTP injection, he cried inconsolably for an entire night. I will never forget trying to comfort my four-month-old baby and being so frightened and helpless. Later, after talking with his pediatrician about the reaction, we went ahead and gave him a new version of the DTP, called DTaP that had fewer side effects. I did not realize that his reaction was a precaution for further vaccines.

One of the other precautions I read for the DTaP vaccine is an "underlying unstable, evolving neurologic disorder." I would consider any child with developmental delay, seizures, ADHD, or autism as having "underlying, unstable evolving neurologic disorders," and parents should be told this is a precaution before vaccination.

Vaccine Side Effects

Vaccines are a medical intervention. With any medical intervention, there are risks and potential side effects. The primary side effects are local skin reactions, such as swelling and redness at the injection site. Low-grade fevers are another common side effect. More serious acute reactions are uncommon, such as seizures, anaphylactic shock, or life-threatening allergic reactions where people stop breathing. For a side effect to be attributed to a vaccine, the reaction must occur soon after the vaccine was given and this has led to some of the controversies surrounding vaccine reactions because some reactions, including severe reactions, may not occur until several days after the inoculation.

The U.S. has a system for the reporting of vaccine reactions. This was established by the *National Childhood Vaccine Injury Act* passed by Congress in 1986. It is a centralized vaccine reaction reporting system called *VAERS (Vaccine Adverse Event Reporting System)*, which is jointly operated by the FDA and the CDC. The vaccine injury act requires doctors and vaccine providers to report serious health problems from vaccines. However, it is estimated that 10% or even less of adverse vaccine reactions are actually reported (www.nvic.org). Parents can also report reactions. Although I knew about the system when my son had his reaction, neither my son's pediatrician nor I ever reported it.

Although many reactions are not reported, there have been enough serious reports that have led to over 2 billion dollars being awarded in compensation by the federal government to children and adults injured by vaccines (www.nvic.org). Many families' claims have been rejected, and I know personally some families of children with autism who have fought for years with no results.

Twelve Crucial Vaccine Issues

Every parent needs to make decisions about vaccinating their child. Should they follow the full schedule? Should they do a modified schedule? Most importantly: are there any individual factors that should be considered? Because of the multiple questions from parents I answer daily and the research I have done, I have assembled twelve individual issues a family should consider and discuss with their child's health practitioner before beginning a vaccine schedule for their child.

1. Types of vaccines

Not all vaccines are the same. They are made differently and therefore may cause different reactions.

There are four main types of vaccines:

- *Polysaccharide conjugate vaccines* use sugars from one type of bacteria and bind them to another type of bacteria or virus.
  —Vaccines: HIB (Hemophilus), Pneumococcal, and Menigococcal

- *Killed or inactivated vaccines* use the whole bacteria or virus, but the organism is killed first so it cannot infect a person.
  —Vaccines: IPV (polio), Hep A (Hepatitis A), and Flu (influenza)

- *Live virus vaccines* also use the whole virus, but they are not inactivated.
  —Vaccines: MMR (Measles, Mumps, and Rubella), Varicella (chicken pox), OPV (oral polio) Rotavirus, and Flu (nasal influenza)

- *Genetically engineered vaccines* are made from the DNA of specific viruses. The organisms are grown with yeast cells in order to produce specific proteins.
  —Vaccines: Hep B (Hepatitis B), Gardasil (HPV or human papilloma virus)

The live virus vaccines tend to promote a stronger, more long lasting immune response. Because of this, acute reactions such as fever are more common. If someone's immune system is weakened, they may have more problems with a live virus vaccine. Genetically engineered vaccines are newer, so there is less long-term research about potential complications.

2. Efficacy: do the vaccines work to prevent disease?

Many people think that once vaccines are given, they are 100% effective in preventing a disease and this effectiveness is permanent or lasts a lifetime. However, the level of immunity provided varies with each vaccine.

Most vaccines are given in a series of more than one inoculation at different intervals because one shot is not completely effective. On average, the first dose of a vaccine gives someone 50% immunity. The next dose usually increases the effectiveness to 75% immunity and the third up to 90% immunity. Booster doses are given several years later because the 90% immunity gradually decreases over time. Even among vaccines, there is a different level of immunity after the same number of doses. The pertussis vaccine has an overall lower rate of immunity and a shorter duration of immunity, which is why this vaccine is given repeatedly throughout childhood.[2]

3. Risk of contracting the disease

Some diseases, such as polio, are only found in several developing countries in the world. Unless a person is traveling to one of these countries, or is exposed to an infected person from one of these countries, there is no chance of infection because there is no risk of exposure. For some common diseases, such as rotavirus (which causes diarrhea in young children), the risk of illness may depend on the child's exposure to many other young children. In a daycare setting, disease exposure also depends on the age of the child and the other children at the center. Some illnesses are more commonly seen in specific age groups, and risks for disease vary by age.

4. Risk of serious consequences from the disease

Some diseases have more serious health consequences than others and this should be part of the vaccination decision. We vaccinate for diseases that cause death and paralysis, but we can also vaccinate now for diseases that have little or no long-term health consequences, such as rotavirus. We need to prioritize vaccinations to protect from the diseases that have the most potential to cause greatest harm.

5. Effect on the Immune System
Development of the immune system

Children are not born with a fully developed immune system. During pregnancy, mothers pass immune factors and antibodies to their unborn children. After birth, breastfed children primarily receive immunity from breast milk, which has many antibodies and immune factors that help prevent infection.[3] Because of this, some infections, such as Haemophilus influenzae, are less common in breastfed infants.[4] Children who are bottle-fed develop antibodies after being exposed to infections.

For all infants, the immune system continues to develop on its own over the first few years of life. The innate immune system is the first part of the immune system, and consists of physical barriers such as the lining of the gastrointestinal tract. This part of the immune system is not fully developed until the end of the first year of life.[5] The adaptive immune system provides memory to previous infections in order to prevent infection if the child is exposed to the same infection. This system takes longer to develop.

An immature immune system is why we often see young children with frequent colds and infections. This immature development is also why certain diseases, such as Haemophilus or pneumococcal bacterial infections, are more serious in infants. Therefore, some vaccines are given to young infants because they are at greatest risk for serious infections. However, at the same time, their immune system is not fully developed, and their response to the vaccines may not be optimal or long lasting.

Allergies

The immune system has many components including T-cells, a type of white blood cell. T-cells can be divided into helper T-cells, which help activate the immune system. Helper T-cells can be further divided into Th-1 and Th-2 cells. These two types of helper cells need to be in balance and working together for the immune system to function properly.

Vaccines tend to shift the balance between these two types of helper T-cells, thereby causing an increase in Th-2 cells and a decrease in Th-1 cells. An increase in Th-2 cells tends to increase allergies, asthma, and autoimmune diseases. Therefore, vaccination, especially early, when a child's immune system is not fully developed, may cause an increase in allergies and asthma due to an imbalance of the immune system.[6]

Toxins, such as mercury, lead, and aluminum, also tend to shift the immune system toward an imbalance of too many Th-2 cells, leading to an increase in allergies and asthma. Many children with autism spectrum disorders have problems with allergies, ranging from food and environmental allergies to asthma and eczema.

Autoimmunity

When the body's immune system attacks itself, it is called *autoimmune disease*. The immune reaction can be against any cells in the body from joints in rheumatoid arthritis, to the thyroid in Hashimoto's disease. It has been accepted for decades that an infection can trigger autoimmune disease. A good example is with the bacteria streptococcus that causes strep throat. If left untreated, the strep bacteria can lead to an autoimmune reaction called rheumatic fever. Not everyone who develops strep throat will get rheumatic fever. It appears that some people are genetically more susceptible to autoimmune disease than others.

Since vaccines are made from bacteria and viruses, they also have the potential to lead to autoimmune disease. One of the first associations was made when the swine flu vaccine was given in the 1970s. After the administration of the vaccine, there was an increase in the autoimmune disease called Guillan-Barre syndrome which leads to paralysis of the muscles.[7] The influenza vaccine today still lists the rare development of Guillan-Barre syndrome as a possible side effect.

Children with autism show evidence of autoimmune disease in the brain. Antibodies have been found against myelin and axon filament proteins in the brains of children with autism.[8] Upon researching these autoantibodies in children with autism, a correlation was made between children who had positive antibodies to measles and herpes 6 virus, which causes Roseola.[9,10] In many children with autism, there is also a family history of autoimmune disease.[11]

6. Age of vaccination

Because the immune system is not fully developed during the first few years of life, vaccines given early may not be as effective. In addition, early vaccines may adversely affect immune system development and cause an increased risk of allergies.

Evidence of this can be seen in Japan, where children once received the diphtheria, pertussis, and tetanus (DPT) vaccine at three months of age. Research showed that when the vaccine was delayed until two years of age, there was an 85% to 90% reduction in severe vaccine reactions and deaths.[12] The Japanese government now recommends a range of several years in which to give infants their first immunizations; this includes a new formulation of the DPT vaccine.

Every country recommends a different vaccine schedule for their children, including the type and number of vaccines and the ages when they should be given. Young children in the U.S. receive up to three times as many vaccines as young children in some other countries, and many of these are multiple vaccines given at earlier ages in the U.S. The CDC recommends that children in this country receive their first vaccine the day after they are born!

7. Number of vaccines given simultaneously

The number of vaccines children in the U.S. normally receive has more than doubled in the past two decades. Following the current CDC schedule, by the time a child is six years old, he or she will have received 49 doses of 14 vaccines. An infant at the young ages of two, four, and six months, will receive seven or more vaccines in just one day. Compare these figures to 1983, when a six-year-old child would have received a total of 22 doses. Concern has been raised about the number of vaccines given, especially in the first year of life. A recent research article found a correlation of increased infant mortality with an increased number of vaccines given in the first year.[13] Further research in this area needs to be done since the number of vaccines early in life continues to increase.

When vaccines are tested for reactions, they are given individually, while in practice they are often combined with other vaccines. Some concern has been raised that combining vaccines could lessen the immune response from any one vaccine. This was seen when the Haemophilus influenzae type B (HIB) vaccine was given in a combination vaccine; the antibody response to HIB was lower from the combined vaccine than from a single dose vaccine. We do not know the effects of giving more than one vaccine, much less a combination of multiple vaccines, to a young child with an immature immune system. More thorough testing is needed to ensure the safety of multiple vaccine injections.

8. Ingredients in vaccines

Vaccines contain many ingredients in addition to the bacteria and viruses that are used to make the vaccines. The vaccines need preservatives to prevent contamination from microbes, and adjuvants to increase the effectiveness of the vaccine within the body. The preservative thimerosal and the adjuvant aluminum are of concern. However, less controversial ingredients may also pose a health risk.

Glutamate

Glutamate, a component of monosodium glutamate, is used as a flavor enhancer in food and as a stabilizer in some vaccines. Glutamate is also an excitotoxin. Excitotoxins cause nerve cells to activate and fire impulses, thereby exciting the nervous system. The problem is when the brain starts firing and does not stop. This is not an allergic reaction, but rather a toxic reaction because it harms nerve cells or neurons. As with other toxins, a child's developing nervous system is more at risk to this damage. Glutamate may cause some of the chronic inflammation seen in children with autism, and possibly in other children as well.

Thimerosal

Thimerosal is a preservative added to vaccines since the 1930s. Thimerosal contains 50% mercury in the form of ethylmercury. This is different than the methylmercury form found in fish.

As the number of vaccines given to young children and pregnant women increased in the early 1990s, the amount of mercury exposure also increased. During this same time period, the number of autism cases increased. Because mercury is a known neurotoxin and the fetus in utero and young children are vulnerable, some people made a correlation between the two. Comparisons have been made about the similarities between the symptoms of autism and the symptoms of mercury poisoning, including social impairments, repetitive behaviors, depression, and anxiety.[14] In addition to clinical symptoms, autism and mercury poisoning share similar disruptions in neurotransmitter levels, reductions in immune natural killer cells and T-lymphocytes, glutathione depletion, and increases in the presence of autoantibodies to brain proteins.[15] Acute mercury exposure accidents document the similarity of symptoms. For example, video tapes after the Minomato, Japan accident show children demonstrating behavior seen typically in autism.

Another issue that increased concerns was calculations done on the amount of mercury an infant would receive during the first 6 months of life from the vaccine schedule current in 2001. The total was 200 mcg, which exceeded the EPA's maximal allowable amount.[16] This calculation was based on the EPA recommended limit of 0.1 mcg of mercury per kilogram per day. If an average newborn weighs 7-8 lbs or 3.5 kg, then they should receive no more than 0.35 mcg of mercury per day. Individual vaccines with thimerosal during this time period contained anywhere from 0.3 mcg to 25 mcg per dose. Since multiple vaccines were given on one day, an infant could easily surpass the safe limit of 0.35 mcg per day.

Due to the concerns over thimerosal, as a precautionary measure the American Academy of Pediatrics and the U.S. Public Health Service issued a joint statement in 1999, to remove the thimerosal from vaccines used in children younger than 6 years old.[17] Since 2002, the only vaccine that contains the original amount of thimerosal is inactivated influenza vaccines.

Other current vaccines still contain traces of thimerosal. According to the Immunization Safety Review Committee, the maximum amount of thimerosal mercury that an infant could be exposed to per vaccine is less than 3 mcg per vaccine.[18] While this exposure is much less than before, for a newborn infant 3 mcg per vaccine is still more than the safe amount of 0.35 mcg recommended by the EPA. Again, this is the amount per vaccine and young children receive multiple vaccines on one day, which would increase the overall exposure.

Multiple research studies on the cellular effects of thimerosal have been done since the removal of the preservative in 2002. Research using young rats exposed to thimerosal showed multiple negative effects on brain cells, including damage to nerve cells, and alterations of neurotransmitter levels.[19-22] Several studies found that male animals suffered more severe effects than female animals, which is interesting since we know that autism affects more human males than females.[23,24] Animal research using infant monkeys showed similar negative effects on the brain. These monkeys were given the complete U.S. childhood vaccines used in 1994-1999.[25] Brain scans done on these monkeys showed a decrease in the size of a part of the brain called the *amygdala*.[26]

Fewer studies have been done on humans, although one recently released study did find a correlation between thimerosal-containing vaccines and decreased scores on psychomotor development at 1 and 2 years of life.[27] Conversely, a study that calculated the amount of mercury children were exposed to from vaccines did not find any significant relationship to autism risk.[28] Although no significant statistical correlations were found in this study, upon reviewing the data, it appeared to me that children who had autism with regression received higher amounts of thimerosal prenatally versus children without autism.

Although mercury exposure through thimerosal was decreased by 2002, autism rates have continued to rise. The increase in autism after removal of thimerosal was taken by researchers as evidence that no correlation exists.[29] Critics of the study cite the change in diagnostic criteria for autism and the fact that the autism rates came only from inpatient hospital visits in 1992. Follow-up autism rates were taken from a different population of children from an outpatient clinic. Since a small number of children in general are treated in the hospital, this would lead to a small number of children with autism in the before numbers, compared to the number of children with autism treated in outpatient clinics, leading to a larger overall number of children with autism. Just because overall rates of autism are increasing without thimerosal does not mean that some children were not affected by the mercury in the preservative.

Aluminum

The metal aluminum is used in vaccines as an adjuvant to increase the immune response to vaccines. How this metal enhances immune response is not fully understood. It appears to stimulate the Th2 immune response more than the Th1 response. This means that cytokine chemicals are released to activate the immune system. These chemicals help the vaccine become more effective but also lead to inflammation and oxidative stress. Concern has been raised that people with a genetic tendency toward allergies may be more vulnerable to exaggerated immune responses from the aluminum in vaccines.[30] This exaggerated immune response, which is a TH2 response, may lead to increased allergies and autoimmune issues.[31]

Research studies by the FDA found that daily aluminum levels of greater than 4 to 5 micrograms per kilogram of body weight were associated with damage to the nervous system and bones of infants.[32] For example, 36 micrograms is toxic to a 9-kilogram (20-pound) baby. But many vaccines, such as the hepatitis B vaccine, have 250 micrograms of aluminum per vaccine. And these young children often receive more than one vaccine containing aluminum at a time. Overall, children often receive up to 18 vaccines that contain aluminum. For routine immunization practices at 2 months old for example, children may receive multiple vaccines with aluminum at the same time.

Aluminum is especially toxic to anyone with kidney problems. Although newborns do not routinely have kidney issues, they do have immature kidneys, which may lead to increased problems from injected aluminum.

Based on concerns that aluminum can lead to neurotoxicity and immune stimulation, both of which are primary concerns in autism, researchers tried to evaluate any correlation between aluminum exposure in vaccines and autism prevalence. Results from one study found that countries with the highest autism prevalence appeared to have the highest aluminum exposure from vaccines.[33] In addition, the increase in exposure to aluminum in vaccines over the past two decades parallels the rise in autism over the same time period.[34]

Other substances

Vaccines may contain additional preservatives such as antibiotics or even formaldehyde, a carcinogen. Some vaccines may contain animal tissues, including egg proteins, thereby posing a risk to children with allergies. In addition, yeast, which is an issue for many children with autism, is used as a growth media in some vaccines.

9. Effects of medicines given with vaccines

Tylenol (a form of acetaminophen) is commonly recommended before and after any vaccine to reduce pain and fussiness. However, Tylenol is broken-down in the body into two chemicals, one of which blocks the antioxidant glutathione. Glutathione, part of the liver's main detoxification system, is needed to help detoxify the vaccines. If glutathione is blocked, then a person cannot properly detoxify vaccines, and therefore may have more reactions and problems from vaccines. Although all people will have a decrease in glutathione production from Tylenol, many children with autism have metabolic problems with glutathione depletion and sulfur metabolism, and may have more severe problems with Tylenol because of this.[35] A recent study confirmed this issue. The research showed that children who received Tylenol before the MMR vaccine were more likely to develop autism than children who were not given Tylenol before the vaccine.[36]

Antibiotic use during vaccination is also of concern for similar reasons. If children are on antibiotics, their detoxification system is already working to process the medicine. The vaccines will have to compete with the antibiotics for detoxification, which means that neither the antibiotic nor the vaccine will be detoxified well. Concern has been raised that if children are on antibiotics during vaccination, their bodies will hold onto more of the metals (including mercury and aluminum) used in the vaccines than they would otherwise with resultant negative health effects.

10. Individual ability to detoxify

Glutathione, mentioned above, is just one of multiple detoxification mechanisms in the body. Because there are large differences in individual detoxification abilities, people react to and process vaccines and their ingredients differently.[37,38] The same principle applies to medicines. Some medications work for many people, yet may have no effect on others. Similarly, some people experience medication side effects, while others do not. In considering vaccinations, it is important to consider if a child is sensitive to and has strong reactions to medicines. If they are more reactive, or their parents have a history of poor reactions to medicines, a child may only be able to process one vaccine at a time.

11. Gender

We know that boys have much higher rates of autism than girls. Although no one knows for sure why this difference exists, there is some speculation that the hormones estrogen and testosterone play a role. All boys and girls have both types of hormones, but boys have much more testosterone and girls have much more estrogen. If a parent is vaccinating a boy, they might want to be more cautious, or examine individual and family history more carefully.

12. Personal and family history of vaccine reactions

A child's family history can sometimes give a clue to potential vaccine reactions. It is important to know if anyone in the family has had a severe vaccine reaction. If a parent or a sibling has been affected, I am more concerned about the child in question receiving a vaccine.

One of the parents I work with told me that when she was a child, she stopped breathing after receiving a vaccine. Her one-day-old child also stopped breathing right after her first immunization for hepatitis B. The child's doctor did not attribute the vaccine to the child's incident. However, after the child's first diptheria/tetanus/pertussis (DTaP) vaccine, she had a similar reaction and had to be seen in the hospital. The mother declined further vaccinations for her child, and the child has had no further episodes. She is now a healthy preschool child.

Another important point in the family history is whether anyone in the family has autism. If any siblings have autism, I know that this next child is at higher risk of developing autism. Because of this family history, I am more cautious about vaccinating this next child early in life before I have seen if they are developing normally.

Summary

Vaccine issues to discuss with practitioner

1. Types of vaccines
2. Efficacy: Do the vaccines work to prevent disease?
3. Risk of contacting the disease
4. Risk of serious consequences from the disease
5. Effect on the immune system
6. Age of vaccination
7. Number of vaccines given simultaneously
8. Ingredients in vaccines
9. Effects of other medicines preceding and following vaccinations
10. Individual ability to detoxify
11. Gender
12. Personal and family history of vaccine reactions

Today the standard medical practice is to vaccinate all children with the complete vaccination schedule (a schedule that adds more vaccines every year). While contraindications and side effects are documented on vaccine labels, practitioners rarely perform in-depth reviews of children's health histories, family health histories, and risk factors for the many vaccines. I believe the safest medical practice is for practitioners to review each of the twelve items I describe above with parents to make the healthiest vaccine decisions for their particular child.

REFERENCES CHAPTER 21

1. Institute of Medicine (U.S.) Immunization Safety Review Committee. Immuniza-tion Safety Review: Vaccines and Autism. *Washington (DC): National Academies Press (US);* 2004. DH592.

2. Cherry JD, Brunell PA, Golden GS, Karzon DT. Report of the task force on per-tussis and pertussis Immunization-1988. *Pediatrics* 1988;81 (suppl):9. DH607.

3. M'Rabet L, Vos AP, Boehm G, Garssen J. Breast-feeding and its role in early development of the immune system in infants: consequences for health later in life. *J Nutr.* 2008;138(9):1782S-1790S. DH75.

4. Silfverdal SA, Bodin L, Olcén P. Protective effect of breastfeeding: an ecologic study of Haemophilus influenzae meningitis and breastfeeding in a Swedish popula-tion. *Int J Epidemiol.* 1999 Feb;28(1):152-6. DH608.

5. M'Rabet 2008.

6. Hurwitz HL. Effects of diphtheria-tetanus-pertussis or tetanus vaccination on aller-gies and allergy-related respiratory symptoms among children and adolescents in the United States. *J of Manipulative Physiol Ther.* 2000 Feb;23(2):81-90. DH609.

7. Schonberger LB, Bregman DJ, Sullivan-Bolyai JZ, Keenlyside RA, Ziegler DW, Retailliau HF, Eddins DL, Bryan JA. Guillain-Barre syndrome following vaccination in the National Influenza Immunization Program, United States, 1976--1977. *Am J Epidemiol.* 1979 Aug;110(2):105-23. DH603.

8. Singh VK, Warren RP, Odell JD, Warren WL, Cole P. Antibodies to myelin basic protein in children with autistic behavior. *Brain Behav Immun.* 1993; 7:97-103. DH617.

9. Ibid.

10. Singh VK, Linn SX, Yang VC. Serological association of measles virus and human herpevirus-6 with brain autoantibodies in autism. *Clin. Immunol. Immunopath.* 1998 Oct;89(1):105-108.

11. Comi AM, Zimmerman AW, Frye VH, Law PA, Peeden JN. Familial clustering of autoimmune disorders and evaluation of medical risk factors in autism. *J Child Neurol.* 1999 Jun;14(6):388-94. DH604.

12. Noble, GR, Bernier RH, Esber EC et al. Acellular and whole-cell pertussis vaccines in Japan: Report of a visit by US scientists. *J of the Am Med Association* 1987;257:1351-1356. DH610.

13. Miller NZ, Goldman GS. Infant mortality rates regressed against number of vaccine doses routinely given: is there a biochemical or synergistic toxicity? *Hum Exp Toxicol.* 2011 Sep;30(9):1420-8. DH606.

14. Bernard S, Enayati A, Redwood L, Roger H, Binstock T. Autism: a novel form of mercury poisoning. *Med Hypotheses.* 2001 Apr;56(4):462-71. DH587.

15. Ibid.

16. Ball LK, Ball R, Pratt RD. An assessment of thimerosal use in childhood vaccines. *Pediatrics.* 2001 May;107(5):1147-54. DH589.

17. Thimerosal in vaccines—An interim report to clinicians. American Academy of Pediatrics. Committee on Infectious Diseases and Committee on Environmental Health. *Pediatrics.* 1999 Sep;104(3 Pt 1):570-4. DH591.

18. Institute of Medicine (US) Immunization Safety Review Committee. Immunization Safety Review: Vaccines and Autism. *Washington (DC): National Academies Press (US);* 2004. DH592.

19. Olczak M, Duszczyk M, Mierzejewski P, Meyza K, Majewska MD. Persistent behavioral impairments and alterations of brain dopamine system after early postnatal administration of thimerosal in rats. *Behav Brain Res.* 2011 Sep 30;223(1):107-18. DH593.

20. Duszczyk-Budhathoki M, Olczak M, Lehner M, Majewska MD. Administration of thimerosal to infant rats increases overflow of glutamate and aspartate in the prefrontal cortex: protective role of dehydroepiandrosterone sulfate. *Neurochem Res.* 2012 Feb;37(2):436-47. DH594.

21. Olczak M, Duszczyk M, Mierzejewski P, Wierzba-Bobrowicz T, Majewska MD. Lasting neuropathological changes in rat brain after intermittent neonatal administration of thimerosal. *Folia Neuropathol.* 2010;48(4):258-69. DH595.

22. Olczak M, Duszczyk M, Mierzejewski P, Bobrowicz T, Majewska MD. Neonatal administration of thimerosal causes persistent changes in mu opioid receptors in the rat brain. *Neurochem Res.* 2010 Nov;35(11):1840-7.

23. Branch DR. Gender-selective toxicity of thimerosal. *Exp Toxicol Pathol.* 2009 Mar;61(2):133-6. DH597.

24. Olczak 2011.

25. Hewitson L, Lopresti BJ, Stott C, Mason NS, Tomko J. Influence of pediatric vaccines on amygdala growth and opioid ligand binding in rhesus macaque infants: A pilot study. *Acta Neurobiol Exp (Wars).* 2010;70(2):147-64. DH598.

26. Ibid.

27. Mrozek-Budzyn D, Majewska R, Kieltyka A, Augustyniak M. Neonatal exposure to Thimerosal from vaccines and child development in the first 3 years of life. *Neurotoxicol Teratol.* 2012 Nov-Dec;34(6):592-7. DH599.

28. Price CS, Thompson WW, Goodson B, Weintraub ES, Croen LA, Hinrichsen VL, Marcy M, Robertson A, Eriksen E, Lewis E, Bernal P, Shay D, Davis RL, DeStefano F. Prenatal and infant exposure to thimerosal from vaccines and immunoglobulins and risk of autism. *Pediatrics.* 2010 Oct;126(4):656-64. DH605.

29. Madsen KM, Lauritsen MB, Pedersen CB, Thorsen P, Plesner AM, Andersen PH, Mortensen PB. Thimerosal and the occurrence of autism: negative ecological evidence from Danish population-based data. *Pediatrics.* 2003 Sep;112(3 Pt 1):604-6. DH586.

30. Terhune TD, Deth RC. How aluminum adjuvants could promote and enhance non-target IgE synthesis in a genetically-vulnerable sub-population. *J Immunotoxicol.* 2012 Sep 11. DH600.

31. Tomljenovic L, Shaw CA. Mechanisms of aluminum adjuvant toxicity and auto-immunity in pediatric populations. *Lupus.* 2012 Feb;21(2):223-30. DH601.

32. Bishop, NJ, Morley R, Day JP, Lucas A. Aluminum neurotoxicity in preterm infants receiving intravenous feeding solutions. *NEJM.* 1997;336(22):1557-1561. DH613.

33. Tomljenovic L, Shaw CA. Do aluminum vaccine adjuvants contribute to the rising prevalence of autism? *J Inorg Biochem.* 2011 Nov;105(11):1489-99. DH602.

34. Ibid.

35. Waring RH, Klovrza LV. Sulphur Metabolism in Autism. *Journal of Nutritional & Environmental Medicine.* 2000. 10:25-3. DH590.

36. Schultz ST, Klonoff-Cohen HS, Wingard DL, Akshoomoff NA, Macera CA, Ji M. Acetaminophen (paracetamol) use, measles-mumps-rubella vaccination, and autistic disorder: the results of a parent survey. *Autism.* 2008 May;12(3):293-307.

37. Gonzalez FJ, Gelboin HV. Role of human cytochrome P-450s in risk assessment and susceptibility to environmentally based disease. *J Toxicol Environ Health.* 1993 Oct-Nov;40(2-3):289-308. DH611.

38. Allorge D, Loriot MA. Pharmacogenetics or the promise of a personalized medicine: variability in drug metabolism and transport. *Ann Biol Clin* (Paris).2004;62(5):499-511. DH612.

Conclusion

As autism and ADHD have become increasingly common, they are exacting a tremendous toll on individuals, families, and society. We can no longer sit by and watch as the health of our children is compromised.

Thanks to researchers, we now know dozens of risk factors that encompass the areas of nutrition, digestion, metabolism, immunity, and environmental toxins. It makes sense that if we address these risk factors, we will reduce the occurrence of these diseases.

It is time to educate women that their health and their baby's health are intertwined. We need to show women that their baby's health depends on them even before conception. A mother who prepares herself for pregnancy has the opportunity to reduce her child's risk of developing autism and ADHD.

❖❖❖

Throughout this book, I have raised issues that need to be addressed to improve the health of our children. Below I have summarized these issues with the intent that people can move forward after reading this book and become child health advocates themselves.

Supporting Effective Autism and ADHD Treatment

Modern medicine has its strengths and its challenges. It works best in acute trauma care situations. In a car accident the diagnosis and course of treatment is clear: the broken limb needs to be fixed and the laceration needs to be sutured.

Modern medicine stumbles when presented with multiple symptoms and no single cause. Such is the case with autism and ADHD. Chronic diseases are now more and more common in children and child healthcare providers need to adjust to the needs of these children.

My patients with autism present with limited or no speech and poor sociability—the common signs of autism. But they often have abdominal pain, seizures, allergies, poor muscle tone, and skin rashes. Modern medicine cannot effectively treat an array of symptoms like these in the normal 10-minute pediatric visit. This leaves parents to search on their own for health care practitioners who will to spend the needed to time to unravel and treat the multitude of health issues these children have.

This situation needs to change. Heath insurers and government policy makers need to recognize autism and ADHD as medical, not psychological diseases and cover the costs of needed treatment. We must support doctors and other therapists who make the decision to care for these children.

The CDC and Prevention

Research funding from the CDC into autism and ADHD has focused on discovery of genetic causes and various risk factors. The CDC states that the causes of autism are elusive but are most likely a combination of genes and the environment.

Our country stepped up for heart disease prevention. Patients are advised to exercise, control stress and eat better. Patients review their family history for heart attacks.

How long will the CDC focus solely on the epidemiology of autism and ADHD before realizing that the implementation of preventative programs could dramatically reduce the incidence of these diseases in the first place? How many risk factors need to be discovered before it makes the decision that programs are needed to educate women how to reduce their particular risk factors?

It seems that prevention is not currently at the forefront of the CDC agenda on autism and ADHD. The name "Centers for Disease Control" is actually a little longer. The full name of the CDC is "Centers for Disease Control and Prevention." It is time for the CDC to allocate funding for research and education to prevent autism and ADHD.

Autism and ADHD Prevention Programs

What would an autism and ADHD prevention program look like? Family physicians, obstetricians, midwives and other health care professionals would receive training so they can educate women for better preconception and maternal health. Education materials need to be developed that clearly illustrate the mother-child health combination and how to strengthen and protect this bond. Women need to be informed about their options so they can make the best decisions around the time of birth. The trend of increasing voluntary C-sections needs to be reversed.

Individualized Vaccines

Vaccination practices need to be decided based upon the risks and benefits to the particular mother and child. There may be more contraindications for particular vaccines than is currently practiced in this country. Both family history and individualized histories need to be evaluated fully in order to make the best-informed choices for each patient.

Canaries in a Coal Mine

Before the time of automated air quality monitoring, miners used to take canaries with them deep into their mines. If the bird became ill, the miners knew that air quality was poor and to immediately leave that section of the mine. The canary was more vulnerable than the miners and showed symptoms of poor air quality that did not yet affect the miners.

The fetus and infants are our canaries. They are tiny compared to adults and are affected by toxins that do not affect full-grown women. The increasing diseases of autism, ADHD, asthma, and allergies in our children are telling us adults that our environment is increasingly toxic. The increase in chemicals and plastics has been so slow as to hardly be noticed, but these substances are now ever-present. The exposure to phthalates, parabens, and a plethora of other chemicals is increasing yearly. Diseases in our children show the result.

Increasing use of plastics and other chemicals is associated with this time of exploding autism and ADHD rates. But individual companies and industries have massive influence on government and the EPA is challenged to provide clear policy and enforceable regulations that would reduce toxin exposure in this country.

The EPA's mission is to protect people and the environment. The low level but continuous exposure to toxins is creating major health crisis seen in increasing childhood diseases like autism. It is time for the EPA to step up to the plate and for voters and health professionals to let our government know about the changes that need to be made for better child health.

The Precautionary Principal

In the U.S., a product is deemed safe until it is proven unsafe. It is difficult to prove a product is unsafe unless its toxic effects are immediate and obvious. The problem in this country is the cumulative effect of all the low level toxins and how multiple chemicals interact with one another.

The fetus is especially vulnerable to toxins. Studies show that there are particular windows of susceptibility to toxins, such as when the neural tube is being formed. A mother needs to protect her child from known hazards, but also needs to be precautionary by protecting her child from unconfirmed hazards. Will EMFs (such as from cell phones) turn out to be harmful to a developing fetus? We don't know. If they turn out not to be harmful, a precautionary woman will simply be inconvenienced. If, however, it turns out that EMFs are harmful to the fetus, a precautionary woman would have avoided a major health issue in her child.

The European Union bans substances not proven to be safe. America should adopt this practice.

Sun, Food, and Antibiotics

Prospective mothers, pregnant women and young children need more sunlight. Sun avoidance recommendations have resulted in chronically low levels of vitamin D. We know that vitamin D has many positive health effects and that it even acts like a hormone.

We need more widely available and cheaper organic food. Pesticides on conventionally grown food are incredibly harmful to a fetus' developing nervous system. Hormones added to our food supply are causing disturbing health problems that disproportionally affect our boys.

Overuse of antibiotics has destroyed the gut flora of many of our children. This compromises their immune system leading to a circle of infections, more antibiotics, and more infections. Childhood infections should be closely monitored by parents under the supervision of their physician. If the infection presents as bacterial, then an antibiotic may be needed. However, in most cases the infection will be viral and no antibiotic is necessary. This one change of practice would reap tremendous health benefits for our children.

Thank you for reading this book. I hope this has been an educational journey and that it will help you make positive changes for what we value most: the health of our children and our future children.

For More Information

For additional resources for improving child health starting before pregnancy, including: healthier products, links to other organizations, books, government websites, lists of healthy choices, and links to Dr. Hamilton's medical practices, see:

PreventingAutismADHD.com

Acknowledgements

First, I would like to acknowledge and thank my amazing, hard-working husband, Mark Baker, who has spent countless hours as research assistant, editor, and book designer. This book would never have been completed without his unwavering support and dedication.

Kristina Ivic designed the beautiful cover. Noah Shannon provided key editorial guidance. John Blakeslee and Veronica Baker were excellent editors. Betty Taylor helped with the book layout. Janamarantha Cote proofread the book. And Josh Mazer's research and parent perspecitve was invaluable.

Finally, I would like to thank my family and friends: Pat Baker, Betsy Hamilton, Marshall Hamilton, Aleah Horstman, Keith Horstman, Sandy Levy, and Greg Wells.

Acronyms

AA - Arachidonic acid
AAP – American Academy of Pediatrics
ABS - Acrylonitrile/butadiene/styrene (Styrofoam™)
ACOG - American Congress of Obstetricians and Gynecologists
ADHD – Attention Deficit and Hyperactivity Disorder
ALA - Alpha-linolenic acid
ALS - Amyotrophic Lateral Sclerosis
ALT - Alanine aminotransferase
ASD – Autism Spectrum Disorder
AST - Aspartate aminotransferase
BHA - Butylated hydroxyanisole
BHT - Butylated hydroxytoluene
BPA - Bisphenol A
BRAT - Bread, rice, applesauce, and toast
BzBP - Benzyl piperazine
CBC - Complete Blood Count
CDC – Centers for Disease Control and Prevention
CDSA - Complete digestive stool analysis
CFL – Compact florescent lightbulb
CFU - Colony-forming units
CHARGE - Childhood Risks from Genetics and the Environment
CIR - Cosmetics Ingredients Review
CO2 - Carbon dioxide
CPSC - Consumer Product Safety Commission
CSC - Campaign for Safe Cosmetics
DBP - Dibutyl phthalate
DDT - Dichlorodiphenyltrichloroethane
DEA - Diethanolamine
DEHP - Di[2-ethylhexyl] phthalate
DEP - Diethyl phthalate
DHA - Docosahexaenoic acid
DINP - Diisonony phthalate
DMP - Dimethyl phthalate
DMPS - 2,3-dimercapto-propanesulfonate
DMSA - Dimercaptosuccinic acid

DNA - Deoxyribonucleic acid

DPT - Diphtheria, pertussis, and tetanus vaccine

DTaP - Diptheria, tetanus, and pertusses vaccine

DTP - Diphtheria, tetanus, and pertussis vaccine

EDSTAC - Endocrine Disruptor Screening and Testing Advisory
        Committee

EDTA - Ethylenediaminetetraccetic acid

EEG - Electroencephalogram

EKG - Electrocardiogram

EMF - Electromagnetic fields

EPA - Eicosapentaenoic acid

EPA – Environmental Protection Agency

ETOH - Alcohol

EU - European Union

EWG - Environmental Working Group

FAS - Fetal Alchohol Syndrom

FDA – Food and Drug Administration

GABA - Gamma-aminobutyric acid

GLA - Gamma-linolenic acid

GM - Genetically modified food

GMO - Genetically modified organism

HCl – Hydrochloric acid

HDPE - High density polyethylene

HIB - Haemophilus influenzae type B

HIV - Human Innunodeficiency virus

HPV - Human papillomavirus

IAOMT - International Academy of Oral Medicine and Toxicology

IgA - Immunoglobulin A

IgE - Immunoglobulin E

IgG – Immunoglobulin G

IBD - Irritable Bowel Disease

IBS – Irritable Bowel Syndrome

IOM - Institute of Medicine

IU - International unit

IV - Intravenus

LA - Linolenic acid

LDPE - Low density polyethylene

MMR - Measles, mumps, and rubella vaccine
MRSA - Methicillin resistant staph aureus
MSG - Monosodium glutamate
MSM - Methylsulfonylmethane
MTHFR - Methylenetetrahydrofolate reductase
NHNES - National Health and Nutrition Examination Survey
NIEHS - National Institute of Environmental Health Sciences
NIH - National Institutes of Health
NRDC - National Resources Defense Council
NSAID - Non-steroidal anti-inflammatory drugs
OAT - Organic acid test (urine)
ORV - Oral polio vaccine
PANDAS - Pediatric autoimmune disease associated with strep
PBDE - Polybrominated diphenyl ether
PCB - Polychlorinated biphenyl
PDD-NOS - Pervasive developmental disorder -- not otherwise
        specified (no longer preferred)
PEG - Polyethylene glycol
PETE - Polyethylene terephalate
PHS - Public Health Service
PMS - Pre-menstrual syndrome
PPD - P-phenylenediamine
PVC - Polyvinyl chloride
RBC - Red blood cell
RNA - Ribonucleic acid
SAD – Standard American Diet
SIDS - Sudden infant death syndrome
SPF - Skin protective factor
Tdap - Tetanus, diptheria and pertussis vaccine
TEA - Triethanolamine
TORCH - Toxoplasmosis, other, rubella, cytomegalovirus, and
        herpes
TRH - Thyrotropin-releasing hormone
TSH - Thyroid-stimulating hormone
UV - Ultraviolet
UVA - Ultraviolet A
UVB - Ultraviolet B

VAERS - Vaccine Adverse Event reporting System
VOC - Volitile organic chemicals

Index

A

AA 71
AAP 232, 233, 241, 272
ABS 133
Acetaminophen 174, 203, 204, 275
Acetic acid 219
Acetone 162
Acetylation 172
Acetylcholine 161
Acetyl-glutathione 177
Acid blocker 89, 90, 244, 245
Acid reflux 80
Acne 89
ACOG 195
Acrylonitrile 132
Acupressure 205
Acupuncture 113, 119, 205
Adaptogenic 113
ADHD
  Hyperactivity 56
  Iron 66
  Pitocin 220
  Rates 2
  Smoking 12
  Toxins 26, 158
Adrenal
  Exhaustion 110, 111
  Hormones 41, 109, 115, 201
  Insufficiency 110, 113
  Stress 110, 111
Advil 204
Aggression 151, 162
Air pollution 139
ALA 71
Alcohol 125, 188, 200
Aldosterone 109
Allergen 86
Allergic reactions 224, 265
Allergy 10, 24, 50, 57, 69, 94, 101,
    111, 239, 255, 269, 274, 275
Aloe vera 85
Aluminum 152, 262, 274, 275

Alzheimer's disease 59, 152
Amino acid 54, 114
Ammonia 162
Amoxicillin 204
Amygdala 273
Amyotrophic lateral sclerosis 59
Anaphylactic shock 57, 265
Anemia 66, 218
Anesthesia 220, 222
Angelman's syndrome 13
Animal study 17, 55, 108, 135, 159,
    160, 161, 162, 203, 255, 273
Antibiotics 24, 46, 47, 81, 84, 86,
    89, 204, 221, 223, 224, 244,
    245, 275
Antibodies 93, 94, 95, 98, 99, 268
Antidepressants 188
Anti-fungals 101
Antimony 151
Antioxidant 59, 151
Antiperspirant 152
Anxiety 59
Apgar score 218
Arching 236, 247
Arsenic 14, 125, 151
Aspartame 54
Aspartic acid 54
Aspirin 204
Asthma 11, 56, 57, 70, 83, 94, 95,
    126, 187, 269, 283
Astragalus 99
Autism
  Cause xi, 5, 9–16, 282
  Costs 4
  Definition 2, 4
  Heavy metals 26
  Nutrition 51
  Prevention 5, 6, 17, 19, 21, 28, 29,
    72, 90, 242
  Rates 1
  Risk factors. *See* Risk factors
  Symptoms 21, 22, 67

246
Protruding eyes 115
Prozac 204
Psychomotor development 273
Puberty 48

Q

Quercetin 102

R

Radiation 116, 127
Ranitidine 204
Rashes 97, 129
Reasoning ability 72
Red raspberry 204
Reflux 24, 80, 85, 89, 90, 236
Renal system 128
Research 16, 17, 28, 40
Rett syndrome 13
Rheumatoid arthritis 10, 94
Rhogam 212
Rice 237
Rickets 234
Risk factors 9, 10, 10–12, 11, 17, 19,
    21, 27, 42, 47, 64, 84, 93, 95,
    96, 111, 115, 132, 139, 147,
    158, 212, 217, 219, 232, 242
  Environmental 14, 16, 40
  Family history 10
Roman chamomile 254
Roseola 95, 270
Rotavirus 266, 267
Rubella 96, 213, 266

S

Sage 235
Salicylates 56
Salmonella 82
Sauna 185
S Boulardii 86, 248
Seafood 146, 199–200
Seeds 65, 73
Seizures 5, 59, 265

Selenium 94, 118
Sensory processing 26
Serotonin 138, 201
Sertraline 204
SIDS 255
Silicone 256
Simethicone 247
Skin 68, 102, 128, 172
  Care 252–254
  Lightener 163
  Skin cancer 70
Small bowel bacterial overgrowth
    81
Smith-Lemli-Opitz syndrome 13
Smog 136
Smoking 187–188
Socialization 72
Sodium benzoate 57
Sodium laureth sulfate 159
Solvents 136, 137, 162, 187
Soy 235
Speech 2, 3, 5, 12, 21, 72, 115, 146,
    282
Sperm 135, 138, 157, 182
Spina bifida 64
Spinal cord 40, 220, 222
Spitting up 236
Steroid 102
Steroid hormones 109, 118
Stinging nettles 102
Stomach 80, 85
  Pain 57
Stool test 86
Strep 223, 269
Stress 4, 11, 15, 16, 42, 46, 56, 80,
    89, 94, 99, 100, 101, 107–
    112, 234
Stretch marks 68
Styrene 136
Styrofoam 133, 134
Sucralose 54
Sugar xiv, 48, 50, 51–53, 86, 99,
    176, 202
Sulfation 172

262, 263, 266
Vision 26
Vitamin 39, 64, 94
Vitamin A 73
Vitamin B 112
Vitamin B6 205
Vitamin B12 39, 64, 75, 173, 177,
    198
Vitamin C 87, 99, 102, 112, 197
Vitamin D 64, 65, 69–71, 99, 165,
    199, 233
Vitamin E 51
Vitamin K 224
VOC 255, 257

W

Water 48, 49
Weight gain 195
White blood cells 95
Whole food 48
Whooping cough 213
Wireless network 211

X

Xenoestrogens 119, 126
X-ray 127, 210
Xylene 136, 255

Y

Yeast 47, 52, 75, 81, 84, 85, 86, 89,
    96, 100, 275
Yoga 112

Z

Zantac 80, 204, 245
Zeolite 148
Zinc 51, 57, 59, 64, 65, 67–69, 76,
    99, 150, 164, 188, 197, 233,
    237, 243, 244
Zinc oxide 164
Zoloft 204